Praise for *The Warrior Diet*

"In my quest for a lean, muscular body, I have seen practically every diet and suffered through most of them. It is also my business to help others with their fat loss programs. I am supremely skeptical of any eating plan or "diet" book that can't tell me how and why it works in simple language. Ori Hofmekler's *The Warrior Diet* does just this, with a logical, readable approach that provides grounding for his claims and never asks the reader to take a leap of faith. *The Warrior Diet* can be a very valuable weapon in the personal arsenal of any woman."

—**DC Maxwell, 2-time Women's Brazilian Jiu-Jitsu World Champion, Co-Owner, Maxercise Sports/Fitness Training Center and Relson Gracie Jiu-Jitsu Academy East**

"The credo that has served me well in my life and that which I tell my patients is that I only take advice from those who practice what they preach. To me, there is nothing more pathetic and laughable than to see the terrible physical condition of many of the self-proclaimed diet and fitness experts of today. Those hypocrites who do not live by their own words are not worth your time, or mine.

At the other extreme, Ori Hofmekler is the living, breathing example of a warrior. There is real strength in the sinews of his muscle. There is wisdom and power in his words. His passion for living honestly is intense and reflective of the toil of a tough army life. Yet in a fascinating and true Spartan way, his physical nature is tempered by an equal reveling in the love of art, knowledge of the classic poets, and in the drinking of fine wine with good conversation.

Welcome *The Warrior Diet* into your life and you usher in the honest and real values of a man who has truly walked the walk. He has treaded the dirt of the path that lay before you, and is thus a formidable guide to a new beginning. He is your shepherd of integrity that will lead you out of the bondage of misinformation. His approach is what I call "revolutionarily de-evolutionary". In other words, your freedom from excess body fat, flat energy levels, and poor physical performance begins with unlearning the modern ways, which have failed you, and forging a new understanding steeped in the secret traditions of the ancient Roman warrior."

—**Carlon M. Colker, M.D., F.A.C.N., author of *The Greenwich Diet*, CEO and Medical Director, Peak Wellness, Inc.**

"I refuse to graze all day, I have better things to do.
I choose *The Warrior Diet*."

—**Pavel Tsatsouline, author of *Power to the People!* and *The Russian Kettlebell Challenge***

"*The Warrior Diet* certainly defies so-called modern nutritional and training dogmas. Having met Ori on several occasions, I can certainly attest that he is the living proof that his system works. He maintains a ripped muscular body year round despite juggling extreme workloads and family life. His take on supplementation is refreshing as he promotes an integrated and timed approach. *The Warrior Diet* is a must read for the nutrition and training enthusiast who wishes to expand his horizons."

—Charles Poliquin, author of *The Poliquin Principles* and *Modern Trends in Strength Training*, Three-Time Olympic Strength Coach

"Despite its name, *The Warrior Diet* isn't about leading a Spartan lifestyle, although it is about improving quality of life. With a uniquely compelling approach, the book guides you towards the body you want by re-awakening primal instinct and biofeedback—the things that have allowed us to evolve this far.

"Ironically, in a comfortable world of overindulgence, your survival may still be determined by natural selection. If this is the case, *The Warrior Diet* will be the only tool you'll need."

—Brian Batcheldor, Science writer/researcher, National Coach, British Powerlifting Team

"Ori Hofmekler has his finger on a deep, ancient and very visceral pulse—one that too many of us have all but forgotten. Part warrior-athlete, part philosopher-romantic, Ori not only reminds us what this innate, instinctive rhythm is all about, he also shows us how to detect and rekindle it in our own bodies. His program challenges and guides each of us to fully reclaim for ourselves the strength, sinew, energy and spirit that humans have always been meant to possess."

—Pilar Gerasimo, Editor in Chief, *Experience Life Magazine*

"In a era of decadence, where wants and desires are virtually limitless, Ori's vision recalls an age of warriors, where success meant survival and survival was the only option. A diet of the utmost challenge from which users will reap tremendous benefits."

—John Davies, Olympic and professional sports strength/speed coach

"I think of myself as a modern-day warrior; businessman, family man and competitive athlete. In the 2 years that I have been following *The Warrior Diet*, I have enjoyed the predators' advantage of freedom from the necessity of frequent feedings. I also benefit from the competitive edge of being a fat burning machine. My 12-year-old son, who is also a competitive athlete, has naturally gravitated towards *The Warrior Diet*. He is growing up lean, strong and healthy, unlike many of his peers, many of whom, even in this land of plenty, are overweight and frequently sick. Thank you, Ori, for writing *The Warrior Diet*."

—Stephen Maxwell, Ms., 2-time Brazilian Jiu-Jitsu World Champion, Co-Owner, Maxercise Sports/Fitness Training Center and Relson Gracie Jiu-Jitsu Academy East

"At a certain age, I began to notice a change in my pre-competition training. The intense physical stress I put my body under started to leave me feeling burnt out after my workouts. I also suffered from frequent sugar crashes due to my Hypoglycemia.

I would become irritated, light-headed and physically weak. I often became angry after training and I could not explain why. I was having a difficult time trying to figure out what and when to eat. This became a serious problem. Competing on an international level, proper diet and training are the bare necessities for peak performance.

After meeting Ori he advised me on what and when to eat. Once I modified my diet my energy levels changed immediately. I was able to work harder through out my workouts. I no longer felt total fatigue after training. Ori and I are of one mind when it comes to functional training. In Martial Arts you must train every aspect of movement in order to perform well. Ori's advice had a direct effect on the way I trained for my two international titles this year.

The information in *The Warrior Diet* will help you achieve the next level in training for the 21st century. It is the physical training along with the diet that will make a lasting impact on your life. I am deeply grateful for Ori's advice and the friendship we have established over the years."

—Sifu John R. Salgado, World Champion, Chinese Wrestling and Taiji Push Hands

"Ori and I became friends and colleagues in 1997 when he so graciously took me under his wing as a writer for *Penthouse* Magazine and *Mind and Muscle Power.*

When I received *The Warrior Diet* in the mail I nearly burst with pride. Not only because my dear friend had finally reached his particular goal of helping others be the best they can be physically, but because I had a small role in the creation of the book. Ori enlisted my help in researching topics such as the benefits of fasting, the perfect protein, and glycogen loading. I believe in Ori's concepts because I trust him wholeheartedly and because I helped uncover the scientific data that proves them. I also live by *The Warrior Diet,* although not to the extreme that Ori does. My body continues to get tighter and more toned in all of the right places...and people marvel at my eating practices.

Read *The Warrior Diet* with an open mind. Digest the information at your own pace. Assimilate the knowledge to make it fit into your current lifestyle. You will be amazed at how much more productive and energetic you will be. Be a warrior in your own right. Your body will thank you for it."

—Laura Moore, Science writer, *Penthouse* **Magazine,** *IronMan* **Magazine, Body of the Month for IronMan, Sept 2001, Radio Talk Show Host** *The Health Nuts,* **author of** *Sex Heals*

THE
WARRIOR
DIET

ORI HOFMEKLER
With Diana Holtzberg

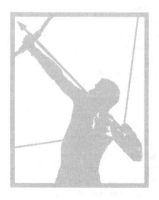

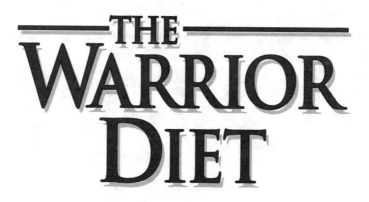

THE WARRIOR DIET

ORI HOFMEKLER
With Diana Holtzberg

Published in the United States by:
Dragon Door Publications, Inc
P.O. Box 4381, St. Paul, MN 55104
Tel: (651) 487-2180 • Fax: (651) 487-3954
Credit card orders: 1-800-899-5111
Email: dragondoor@aol.com • Website: www.dragondoor.com

ISBN 0-938045-35-0

Manufactured in the United States
First Edition: January 2002
Book and cover design, Illustrations and photo effects by Derek Brigham
Website http//www.dbrigham.com Tel/Fax: (612) 827-3431 • Email: dbrigham@visi.com
Photographs of the author by Don Pitlik: (612) 252-6797
Photograph of Diana Holtzberg by Anne F. Pollack

DEDICATION

In loving memory of his grandparents Rina and Daniel Hofmekler, I'd like to dedicate this book to my newborn son Nehemiah, to his sisters Nadia and Shira, to his brother Daniel, to his grandparents Ronald and Josephine, and especially to his most beautiful mother, my wife Natasha.

TABLE OF CONTENTS

Chapter Four
What To Consume During
the Undereating Phase

- The Undereating Phase: what to eat—the vital importance of live (raw) foods…the best fruits and vegetables to eat…enzyme-loading for anti-aging…the essential function of probiotics.

- Why minerals are the most important supplements…the best vitamins, antioxidants, herbs, and brain boosters…the *empty-stomach factor* for natural brain boosting.

- The principles of proper protein utilization …creating the correct power-cocktail for maximum vitality and strength …how protein digestion really works…how not to suffer from allergies, inflammation, water retention, gas, and other digestive disorders.

- Why protein powders can be superfoods—or a nutritional gun to your head…whey proteins, growth factors, immunosupportive factors…why commercial whey proteins can be useless, if not downright dangerous.

- Dairy protein powders—distinguishing the safe from the deadly…several reasons not to use soy protein powders…when and how to use egg-protein…Lactoferin, the magic bullet for immune support.

- The role of carbohydrates during the Undereating Phase—what you can and can't eat.

- Summary of the Undereating Phase—from deep-cleanse detox to a fat-burning army-of-one.

Chapter Five
The Overeating Phase

- How to consume all the food you want—without gaining a smidgen of body fat.

- The Overeating Principles…the three rules of eating…the goals of overeating…how to accelerate your anabolism for tissue repair and building muscles…boosting your metabolism and replenishing essential glycogen…retraining to eat instinctually.

- The science of controlled overeating…exploring the advantages of overeating…the metabolic factor of high-calorie meals…how to make bingeing your happy slave…when to eat carbs if you want to drop fat.

- The crucial importance of *subtle taste*—how to get it back if you've lost it...how to beat the craving for fast-food meals.
- The golden rules of overeating...the secret to instinctively eating the right amount, and knowing when to stop eating—every time.

- The advantages of eating cooked, warm food...triggering the Predator Instinct...Napoleon and the Predator Instinct.
- Vegetables: Cooking vegetables to optimize nutrients and flavors...potentiating flavones to protect against stubborn fat and cancer...the value of soups and stews.
- Protein: Meat, poultry, and fish—for higher testosterone and sperm count...the importance of organic food...deficiency dangers for vegetarians...eggs, yolk and white—when, why and how... the best sources of dairy protein...whey protein... Warrior Growth Serum and Warrior Milk...legumes, beans, and peas—the gladiator protein...the aphrodisiac effect of beans...the ancient—and best—way to prepare beef, fish, and fowl...rotating protein to avoid allergies.
- Fat: Yes/no/maybe—the true skinny on oil and fat use...the must-have, essential fatty acids...the infallible smell test...put the brakes on aging with lipase—nature's natural fat-smasher...the surprising dangers of polyunsaturated oils/fatty acids...hydrogenated and saturated oils—butter: yes, margarine: no, cocoa butter: yes.
- Nuts and seeds—how to consume all you want and even lose weight...almonds—the greatest nut...potent aphrodisiac and secret cancer-killer...peanuts—the good, the bad, and the ugly news...when and how to eat seeds...the value of lecithin.
- Carbohydrates: Knowing your carbs—optimal preparation strategies...when to eat carbs for fat loss...carbs for sounder sleep...controlling your insulin by manipulating the glycemic index...the safest carbs...why to minimize fruits at the main meal...barley—the gladiator grain...why wheat is the least desirable grain...the benefits of sprouted wheat...the magic of chewing dry cereal.

- Sweet meals for "sweet tooths"...when it's safe to indulge in a sweet dessert...meals—for better fat loss...fiber to reduce cholesterol and protect against cancer.
- Fermented foods to aid digestion and optimize metabolism...eliminating yeast infections...enhancing protein uptake for athletes...the pros and cons of vinegar...the pros and cons of wine.
- How to control your acid-alkaline balance...understanding the secret pitfalls of the glycemic index...the dangers of salt restriction...balancing your sodium-potassium pump...the best salts to consume.
- The most allergenic foods—how to avoid sensitivities and allergies.
- What is not allowed on the Warrior Diet...what absolutely does not work, never has, and never will.

Chapter Seven
- What is stubborn fat...the three major problems of stubborn fat...what causes stubborn fat...the link to nutrient deficiencies...the age factor...the six things you can do now to avoid stubborn fat.
- How to get rid of stubborn fat...effective natural stubborn fat busters...key anti-aromatase nutrients...why the liver is a key organ in the battle against stubborn fat...the best liver detoxifiers...yohimbe—aphrodisiac, potency weapon and potential fat burner...Warrior's Stubborn Fat Burner: a natural supplement to block estrogen-related stubborn fat...The Warrior Diet—for superb prevention, elimination of stubborn fat.

Chapter Eight
- The problem with unstable diets...the Warrior Diet versus the perils of frequent-feeding.
- Top-selling diets, and how they differ from the Warrior Diet.

Group I: the All-American (Junk Food) Diet, or ultimate "scavenger diet."...the no-win correlation to diabetes, heart attacks, and degenerative diseases...the American "Health Food" diets.

Group II: high-carbohydrate, low-fat, low-protein...the Pritikin and Dean Ornish diets—ineffective for weight loss and a ticket to hypoglycemia, fat phobias, and deprivation.

Group III: The Zone (40/30/30)—some fatal flaws and wrong assumptions....the few plusses and the many minuses.

Group IV: high-protein, low- or no-carbohydrates diets—Atkins, *Protein Power*, and *The Carbohydrate Addict's Diet*... overacidity and imbalance—the Achilles' heel of the Atkins Diet—why chronic deprivation of carbs translates to induced self-misery, self-poisoning, and premature aging...dangerous gimmicks for the desperate.

Group V: holistic diets...Andrew Weil's *Instinctive Healing*...Harvey Diamond's *Fit For Life* series...Macrobiotics—impractical and lacking balance...no freedom, no good...credit and Brownie points for Andrew Weil...but you can do a whole lot better...Harvey Diamond's practical ways to heal yourself—food separation, detox and living foods...some limitations for the active and athletic...the effective breaking of unhealthy habits.

Chapter Nine

- Why 135 lb. Latin warriors were able to conquer the world...what you see is what you get...the Roman concept of physical *cultus*...the idealization of physical appearance... philosophy, spirituality and the warrior's status...the importance of chivalry... key virtues and dangerous vices.

- The Greco-Roman Warrior Cycle—extremes of deprivation and compensation...daytime activities and diet...evening pleasures...the *Cena* and the *Otium*...the Roman concept of food...*crudus*...*humanitas* ...the plebeian diet...basic food preparations...wining and dining in ancient Rome...courses for the evening meal ...carbohydrate content in ancient warrior meals..."high-sky foods"...balancing overindulgence.

- Sickness and medicine...fasting, music and other remedies...Roman health...diet and nutrition...the importance of beans...the role of grains...the commoners' diet...soldiers' meals...living off the land...the ideal Roman diet.

- The functional applications of the Warrior Diet ....the lean physique for survival—fat equals fatal...the relevance of Ramadan...the way of the Mongol...how to live like a warrior in the twenty-first century—and perform at your best physically and mentally.

- Nutritional carbohydrates revisited...carbs as the main source of brain-fuel...how carb deprivation can trigger sugar cravings and massive bingeing surges...carbs, the magnificent stress-blocker...the anti-aging fuel...carbs, the tax-free fuel—and muscle-saving, secret angel...for thyroid control and healthy metabolism.

- Just saying no to chronic carb-depletion...why in-shape, superactive, ancient warriors needed their carbs...recognizing your individual carbo-needs.

Chapter Ten

- The Warrior Diet as a way of life...the different ways of cycling the Warrior Diet...going off the Warrior Diet—and still winning...the awesome addiction to a crisp mind.

- Alternating between the Sympathetic and Parasympathetic Nervous System for maximum metabolic efficiency...the instinctual green light that says yes to overeating...the difference between controlled and uncontrolled overeating...the demonic force of chronic deprivation...how to avoid sudden weight gain... calories per meal not calories per day.

- Why endurance athletes love to stretch their glycogen—how to boost metabolism, build muscles, and lose body fat...how much body fat you need...the dangerous myth of fat storage... why any bulge is a bad bulge...why your body heat doesn't depend on your fat...the true secret of accelerating muscle growth without gaining fat...the vicious whys and wherefores of insulin insensitivity—and the Warrior Diet's natural remedies.

- How to raise the bar of personal freedom using the principles of the Warrior Diet...moving from self-imposed misery to self-directed pleasure.

- The Romantic Instinct—a new definition for romanticism...breaking established rules to build new ones...the relation to humor...breaking societal taboos...false romanticism ...the phony romance of popular rituals—weddings, anniversaries, Valentine's Day...romanticism, love, relationships and beyond.

- The Aggressive Instinct—the positive side of aggression.

- Know the world you live in...an overview of chemical and environmental toxins—and other daily stressors.

- The first and best defense against radioactive, environmental toxins...the power of natural chelation...antiradiation foods, herbs, and nutrients.

- Prostate Cancer—the causes...the bigger truth about DHT...what really creates enlargement of the prostate, or prostate cancer...the role of prolactin... the warrior diet as first defense against prostate-related problems...estrogenic foods and substances to avoid.

- Natural supplements to help alleviate prostate enlargement related symptoms...Pygeum Bark and Saw Palmetto's possible roles in potency and fertility.

- Frequently asked questions by those who have been practicing the Warrior Diet, and by others who are considering it:

- Does exercise influence when and how much you eat?...What if I'm sick?...Should children use this diet?...how to wean kids off sweets and fast food...the Warrior Diet for young adults...How to handle social and business meals while on the Warrior Diet...Can you have nuts or seeds during the Undereating Phase?... What about smoking and alcohol? Are they allowed?

- What to do with all this new energy...If you find it hard to calm down or sleep at night—what you can do.

- The best enzymes to take—and when.

Part Two: The Workout

• Proper breathing to reduce acid-stress, muscle fatigue, stiffness, and exhaustion.

Abdominals

• The prime function of the abdominals...the "Warrior Posture"...triggering maximum contraction...one giant superset for maximum intensity...combining the isometric and isotonic...the best way to work the obliques...how to turn up the heat and keep on cookin'...the crucial importance of the Lower-Back Stretch.

Legs (Knees, Ankles, Calves, Buttocks, Lower Back)

• Activating the joints and maximizing the three factors of strength...pre-exhausting, isolation plus giant superset for maximum pressure and controlled fatigue...how to avoid tendon injuries...the monstrous superset...Front Squats...Back Squats...Hack Squats...Lunges...Sissy Squats—Dynamic Stretching.

Shoulder Exercises

• Why to split shoulder exercises between two workout days...shoulder presses...supersets for antagonistic muscles—pull-ups and shoulder laterals.

Back and Chest Supersets

• Initial superset of Lat Pull-downs and Incline Press for antagonistic-muscle synergy...second superset of Seated Pulley Rows and Flat Bench Press.

• Dead Lifts—how to best activate the most important compound muscle groups and tendons...maximizing waist and back strength.

High-Velocity Training: Explosive Exercises

• When and how to incorporate high-velocity exercises...Clean and Press—the single exercise-of-choice for an effective full-body workout... enhancing agility, and functional strength...Partial-Press reps for greater intensity...going all out with the Clean and Jerk...for maximum gains in strength, endurance, and balance...Frog Jumps...One Leg Jumps.

The Standing Hamstring Stretch

Biceps and Triceps Superset—Combining tricep and bicep exercises into one intense superset.

Warrior Aerobics

• The Warrior aerobic goals...the Warrior aerobic principles.

Warrior Aerobic Exercises

• Why do aerobics before resistance training...getting leaner and tougher...the three factors that affect aerobics...intense aerobics—sprint intervals...accelerating the effect of controlled-fatigue training...when to perform sprint intervals for maximal gains...stationary biking...the cognitive benefits of reading as you ride.

• The Warrior Workout—helping to trigger your Warrior Instinct...how to be light and mighty... performing under pressure...the Workout and the Diet—tips for best results when exercising on an empty stomach.

Women Who Follow the Warrior Workout

• Women's different needs and different priorities...the chance to build a truly functional body... suggestions for women who want to follow the upper-body exercises...building strong, lean, and functional legs without using weights.

Meat Dishes

• Why cooking meats in liquids is healthier than frying, grilling, or baking...combining pleasure with health...*Curry Chicken in Spicy Tomato Broth...Fish and Eggplant in Curry Tomato Sauce*—for rapid weight loss...*Veal and Carrots in Chicken–Tomato Broth.*

Eggs

• Delicious and very nourishing...as high-protein or high-carbohydrate meals...*Egg-White Omelet with Tomato Sauce...Egg-White Omelet with Black Beans...Egg White Omelet with Lentil and Bean Chili...Oatmeal and Eggs...Rice 'n' Eggs...Angel Hair Rice Pasta with Eggs.*

Baked and Grilled Meals

• *Grilled Chicken...Baked Red Snapper.*

Soups

• As appetizers...as the basis for a whole meal...*Potato–Onion Tomato Soup...Miso Soup*—to protect against radioactive pollution and nourish your body with vital minerals.

• How to cook Miso meals (shellfish, fish, or meats).

Desserts

• The great alternatives to sugar-loaded, high-fat, commercial "treats"...how to avoid the sugar-rush and still feel satisfied...Pumpkin Cheesecake—the open invitation to a healthy binge...*Crepe Blintzes...Live Berries Dessert*—the meal with total appeal...*Milk Gelatin...Papaya Gelatin Dessert*—good for digestion and detoxification...Warm Raspberries and Yogurt—a nourishing treat during the Undereating Phase.

Chapter Fourteen
Sex Drive, Potency and Animal Magnetism 293

• Sex, power, and instincts...sex drive and potency as indicators of health and power...animal magnetism—the primal code of male and female attraction...the new standards for success.

• Male performance factors...neuro-health...hormonal balance...vascular health...mental health...the correlation between impotency and chronic diseases...the factor of stress.

• Potency and diet...the correlation between diet, exercise, and hormonal balance...The Pottenger Cat Study—deficient diet and the degradation of species...mass infertility in the modern U.S.

• The syndrome of taking drugs...common medications that can cause impotency—if not coma and death.

• Natural methods to enhance potency...the role of testosterone...which diets, drugs and life-factors affect testosterone production, sex drive and libido...overtraining vs. your sex drive—symptoms to watch for...the impact of aphrodisiac supplements.

- The Warrior Diet's "instinctual living program" for improving potency...experiencing the power of raw living...craving aphrodisiac foods instinctively—the best natural aphrodisiacs and how they can help...satisfying the primal desire for food and sex.

- How and why The Warrior Diet can work as well for women as men...the modern conspiracy against women's bodies...deprivation—the tyranny of current fad diets...the pandemic of obsessions and phobias—a civilization of cultivated discontent.

- Detoxification for rejuvenating all body tissues...live nutrients for fertility, healthy skin, and fat loss...the power of positive bingeing...trusting your feminine instinct.

- Hormonal fluctuations—the link with diet and nutrition...how The Warrior Diet may help with female stubborn fat.

- The personal origin of the Warrior Diet nutritional supplements...how and why supplementation may help...production history...product safety.

The Supplements

- Warrior Growth Serum—the most potent protein powder available today...Warrior Milk—a great supplemental food for accelerating the anabolic process of building muscles...Warrior Greens—a wonderful alkalizer and a potent aid to combat environmental/radioactive toxins...Warrior Probiotics—for the integrity of your gastrointestinal tract flora...Warrior-zyme— a natural way to keep a youthful appearance...as an antioxidant, anti-inflammatory, antiallergenic, and anticancerous agent.

- Warrior Male Performance Support—for enhancing physical performance, mental sharpness, and sexual potency....the natural alternative to dangerous steroids and suspect sex-drugs.

- Warrior Stubborn Fat Burner—alleviating stubborn fat-related problems through three essential factors.
- Warrior Live Minerals—highly ionized coral minerals...essential for correct pH balance... the key role of calcium for health and longevity...as a first defense against radiation.
- Warrior Live Aloe Powder—highly charged base for accelerating mineral absorption...Warrior Premier Norwegian Cod Liver Oil—best natural source of Vitamin D.

THE WARRIOR DIET

FOREWORD

By Harvey Diamond,
author of *Fit For Life*

I met Ori Hofmekler a couple of years ago in a Japanese restaurant. It stunned me how much he ate that night. I had never seen anyone so lean eat like that. At the time, he was editor in chief of *Mind & Muscle POWER* magazine.

I had known of Ori's art for quite a while. His political satirical paintings always struck me as unique, bold, and thought provoking. They are often very funny. His images have stuck in my mind for years. To quote the late, great Joseph Heller, author of *Catch-22* and numerous other classics: "Ori Hofmekler is a painter of great merit with tremendous wit, intelligence, and imagination. He is better at satirical political art than any other artist I know of at this time. His work deserves to be much better known and more widely enjoyed and treasured."

Breaking taboos, exposing lies, and punching holes in political "balloons" are all essential qualities for strong, effective satire. Real satire makes us laugh every time we're shown the naked (and often ugly) truth.

The Warrior Diet isn't satirical art, but the uncompromising integrity of its creator is evidenced here as well. This book is about the art of raw living. I find the concept of *The Warrior Diet* unique, and although it's quite controversial, I believe it will create a revolution in people's lives. *The Warrior Diet* triggers and unleashes primal instincts within us, many of which have been inhibited or dulled. It endorses virtues such as feeling a sense of freedom, alertness, and possessing optimum mental and physical strength. It also redefines what it means to be a warrior, to be tough, and to be romantic. In other words, this isn't just a diet. It's a way of life, a renaissance of the spirit of raw living.

Ori and I share a similar vision. We both believe that detoxification activates a natural self-healing process and should, therefore, be a top priority. We both believe that there is a wisdom is essential for your health, and affects the way you feel. While we naturally have our differences, they do not detract in any way from the overall effectiveness of his approach. Besides, all you have to do is meet Ori and you will quickly see the man is definitely onto something.

While reading Ori's *The Warrior Diet*, I realized that it all makes sense. Concepts such as the Warrior Cycle, the energy cycle— and his explanation of the interplay between materialism and dematerialism— shed new light on how we operate around the circadian clock. Time is an essential factor in the Warrior Diet. Ori calls this "the lost dimension," since the concept of time and cycles doesn't play an important role in most other diets. (My original *Fit For Life* book was based on the circadian clock).

"Unleashing the power of your instincts" is a refrain that appears throughout the book. Ori is at his fascinating best when discussing our human primal instincts, be it the hunter/predator instinct versus the scavenger instinct, the instincts to survive and multiply, or the romantic instinct. Ori demonstrates how each instinct connects to the other and how they all relate to the Warrior Instinct.

This book is akin to a new "manifesto." It covers all aspects of life, including the instinctual connection between food and sex—a connection that penetrates to the core of human existence. Beyond all the unique and intriguing philosophy, vision, and ideas set forth, there is a very clearly defined diet here that I find to be most effective.

"Lessons from History" explains how the Warrior Diet is based on the old traditions of ancient warriors, yet has been updated to be effective for the modern world. It's designed to allow for creativity and individuality, so you can follow its principles in your own unique way.

I find this diet to be as effective for women as it is for men, in spite of all the macho references. As a final note, I believe strongly in "what you see is what you get." Ori is living proof that the Warrior Diet works.

FOREWORD

By Udo Erasmus,
author of *Fats That Heal, Fats That Kill*

The Warrior Diet is an unusual book. It is a book without measurements, but with feeling. A book that encourages you to break rules to find passion. A book not written by academics who anal–yze everything, but by someone who trusts life and questions stupidity, and encourages you to do the same. This alone is reason to read *The Warrior Diet*.

Something in you already knows a lot about how you should live. Find, and listen to, and trust that instinct, author Ori Hofmekler tells you.

Experts have a nasty tendency to make what's natural and simple more complicated. They make their living by collecting rent on the insecurity they create by undermining your common sense. To do that, they snow you with big words.

In that regard, lucky for you, Ori is not an expert. He encourages you to live by an inner wisdom born of 3.5 billion years of development of creatures made from food and for activity—survival, reproduction, discovery, and joy.

You are endowed with a genetic program that knows how to build a healthy body. Do not poison that program with toxic synthetic man-made molecules that have never been present in nature. Provide it with the building blocks it needs to build that body. How do you do that?

Without getting technical, Ori encourages you to get there through interesting information, through tasty recipes for health, through exercise, through lifestyle, through ways of thinking, and through calling the sleeping warrior within you to awake.

Some of my favorite topics:

- Ori's description of the daily sympathetic-parasympathetic rhythm: light food during the day, when energy goes to external pursuits; the big meal in the evening, relaxed with friends, when the day's work is done.

I love the simple logic of it, and it works in practice. Do big meals during the day make you feel lazy? Do light food during waking hours keep you from getting tired while you need alertness for work? Does eating when you're hungry make food taste better? While you read, ask yourself such questions.

- The Warrior Instinct. Whatever you call it, this instinct within us is more reliable than thousands of half-baked rules imposed by half-alive, double blind theoreticians. Rules serve the need to control, but most are out of line with your need for freedom to discover the truths of your own life.

  Your life is a warrior's path. Whether it is to hunt for food, protect your family, village, or country, or to conquer lies and establish truth, the full life has always been a warrior's life.

  The warrior's life involves goals. It has commitment. There is passion. It is heart-felt. It is conscious. You use your creativity. You question, and you build.

  A warrior's life gives expression to the basic, in-built striving to get better. Its confidence comes, not from memorizing, but from doing, observing, examining, arguing, learning, and improving. It is not 9-5, but goes an extra mile or an extra hour, inspired to accomplish goals because they are worthwhile.

- Romanticism: it is much more than a way to get other people to satisfy your sexual urges. It includes that, but also all that you do with passion and care for life.

Rare in books about foods, there is wisdom in the pages of The Warrior Diet. Technicians write most food books, and Ori knows the techniques, but he shows you a possibility—a platform for living your life as well.

Ori's style is easygoing. His sense of history is interesting. His psychology is common sense. His stories are simple and flow. He is flexible, and learns from all his activities. He does not judge.

Ori talks about food, about ambience, about activity (exercise), about friendship, about lifestyle, about romanticism, and provides great recipes.

The Warrior Diet is a book that talks to all of you—the whole person hidden inside. Read the book, think about what he says, try it, find out how it works for you, argue with him if you want, and discover more of who you are.

A Special Note from the Publisher

As Dragon Door's publisher, I'm usually content to lurk behind the scenes. But, in the case of The Warrior Diet, I can't resist jumping in with some personal comments. It deserves a special word, because it's a breakthrough of a book.

The Warrior Diet contains controversial concepts that are bound to rattle some cages in conventional diet circles. Yet, it's clear that there have been few winners in the world of modern diets. Consider weight management, for instance. A new weight-loss program seems to pop out of the woodwork on a daily basis. More Americans today are on diets than in any other time in history, yet more Americans are overweight than ever before. Most diets simply don't deliver. There seems to be some missing ingredient, some fatal flaw that eventually dooms each new diet fad to failure.

Maybe it's time for something genuinely different—not just a tired rehash of the same old shopworn dietisms.

One missing ingredient in modern diets, bluntly put, is that they *lack balls*—and thus they also lack spirit. There's a reason no one seems to know, for sure, what to eat anymore. There's a reason why infertility and impotency rates are at a world-historical high. "To get our balls back", we need to get back in touch with our natural instincts. To regain our spirit, we need to re-engage with our animal zest for life. The Warrior Diet explains why you need to do all this—and it shows you how.

Revolutionary visions most frequently emerge from the crucible of life-experience, rather than traditional book-learning. Mahatma Gandhi was a lawyer, Einstein was a clerk, and Franz Kafka was an insurance salesman. Yet each reached greatness in an area completely different from their "professions." Sometimes what's needed is a person with passion, belief, and personal experience who thinks "out of the box," without being bound to old paradigms that don't work, but still dominate our lives.

I believe that Ori Hofmekler is such a person. A true Renaissance Man, Ori went through Special Forces army training, has been a champion gymnast, a best-selling political artist, and a magazine editor and publisher. He combines formidable training in the physical and martial arts with broad-ranging erudition and a blazing intelligence. His scholarly interests span history, philosophy, literature, art, anthropology and nutritional science.

So, his Warrior Diet is not just about what to eat—the focus of traditional diet books—it's also about how to improve your life. The Warrior Diet represents one man's quest for the Holy Grail of deeply-engaged living. While many of Ori's ideas are startling, they are grounded firmly in history and science. Ori's genius is not only to reveal the secret behind the Roman and Greek warrior's astonishing prowess, but to demonstrate how we can replicate that prowess in modern times.

In The Warrior Diet, Ori teaches us how to trigger the "Warrior Instinct"—so we hunger for life. Ori teaches us to prowl by day—always ready "to pounce and seize." And Ori teaches us to kick back and compensate at night—relaxing, taking pleasure, enjoying our fruits. The miraculous result? A leaner, more muscular body, an enhanced sexual drive, a sharper mind and a healthier, better-looking body.

These are indeed big claims, but the author himself is a living testament to the power of his method. Ori lives his diet—and has the body, mind and energy to prove it. The man is a dynamo. His book is the product of many years of hard research and harder living. It is a wake-up call to all of us who have become tired, confused or disenchanted by the way we eat or live our lives. The Warrior Diet is about maximal engagement in the pleasures of raw living.

You can see I'm excited. This is the reason I'm in publishing—to find and bring you a vision like the Warrior Diet. It's my delight to offer you a book that can genuinely change your life for the better. Such books are few and far between. My suggestion: do the Warrior Diet for six months. And watch what happens *to your body as well as every other area of your life. Ori will be the first to tell you to experiment.* Your mind and body will know what works for you and what doesn't. Once you try the Warrior Diet, I believe you'll find it not only highly effective but also highly enjoyable. Better yet, the Warrior Diet offers what no other diet does—a sense of freedom, of release, of being in touch with life as it was meant to be lived. What more can you ask for?

Ori and I would love to hear from you about your results with the Warrior Diet. Contact us anytime on the **www.dragondoor.com** Discussion Site. Meanwhile, enjoy!

John Du Cane

—John Du Cane
Publisher, Dragon Door Publications

Acknowledgements

I'd like to thank my family, especially my wife Natasha, for all her loving care and advice.

In moments of truth you know who your real friends are. I want to thank Zvika Elgat, the godfather of my newborn son Nehemiah, for his friendship, unconditional love and support. I also want to acknowledge Dr. Carlon Colker and Pavel Tsatsouline for their persistent encouragement.

I'd like to thank Diana Holtzberg for her dedication to this project. Diana's passion and devotion were unyielding. I truly appreciate her assistance in the writing of this book, and for tempering my Israeli accent.

I must also thank Laura Moore, for her generous help with information and research.

A special thanks to John Du Cane, the publisher of The Warrior Diet, for his vital contribution to the creative process, commitment to this project, and for his wisdom, friendship, and encouragement.

I owe thanks to a few others who took part in creating this book project: Michael Maupin for editing, Derek Brigham for sensing the essence of this book and for his unique design, Don Pitlik for his excellent photography, and Dr. Marshall for his contribution to the Warrior Diet Nutritional Supplements.

I'd like to thank Toby Coriell, my associate, for his support and advice when I really needed it.

I'd like to acknowledge the late Bill Lauren, who initially offered to assist me with the writing of The Warrior Diet. Bill was a wonderful writer, and it was my privilege to have worked with him on a health column that I used to edit.

I'd also like to thank all those that follow the Warrior Diet, who send me streams of letters telling me of their progress and testifying that the Warrior Diet really works.

Finally, as strange as it sounds, I'd like to acknowledge my cat Junior. Watching him always gives me inspiration—for his modeling of grace, agility, and instinctual power.

PREFACE

I've been practicing the Warrior Diet on and off for many years.
During this time I've discovered that being on the Warrior Diet
has made me more energetic, alert, instinctive, ambitious, and in
control than those times when I have been off the diet. My
metabolism has accelerated to the point that I find it difficult to
keep my weight from dropping. I'm naturally lean. I don't count
calories, and I eat as much as I want of all the food groups:
protein, fat, and carbohydrates. When sitting at dinner with friends
or family, I used to apologize in advance for the amount of food
that I consume. A few still think that something must be wrong
with me, but by now most of my friends and even some family
members also practice the Warrior Diet. I've heard people say,
"How can anyone eat so much late at night and still be so lean?"
or "It's all genetics," "He is crazy," or "Ori, how come everyone
is finished and you're still eating?" I've noticed that those who are
on weight-loss diets usually enjoy watching others who can eat
unlimited amounts of food. For them, it's a vicarious experience—
a dream come true.

Since "The Warrior Diet" column began running in *Mind &
Muscle Power* magazine, many who have read it, or just heard
about it from others, have been trying to jump in, often without
enough knowledge or information. I've been blitzed with so many
letters and phone calls from people who want advice or guidance
that it became impossible to answer everyone. That is why I've
written this book. Reading it should guide you to practice the
Warrior Diet on your own. This is not just a diet. It's a way of life.
It involves your body and mind, and gives you a sense of
freedom—a sense that, in my opinion, many people lack today.

Hopefully you will find this book intriguing enough to try
practicing my diet plan. If you do, I believe that you'll notice
significant changes in the way you look and feel, and even in the
way you think. It may, in short, change your life.

Those who want information regarding specific food and supplements will find it in the "Undereating Phase," "Overeating Phase," "Warrior Meals and Recipes," and "Warrior Nutritional Supplements" chapters.

The historical component of this book, "Lessons From History," is limited to basic research that shows how the Warrior Diet is actually based on a very old tradition, yet is still very relevant, pertinent, and practical for the twenty-first century.

Life is a struggle. You either win or lose. For a warrior, survival is just not good enough. Warriors want to win. To be a warrior, you don't need a war. All you need is the spirit, which is hidden inside you. This spirit is what I call the "Warrior Instinct." Once unleashed, it will guide you to greater health and your own sense of freedom. And nothing tastes sweeter than freedom.

INTRODUCTION

I'm about to commit dietary heresy. What I'm about to propose will cause an army of doctors, nutritionists, and self-proclaimed dietary experts to wail and gnash their teeth. They'll call me ignorant. They'll read about my revolutionary diet plan—one that can create a society of lean, muscular, modern warriors—and they'll smack their foreheads as they dismiss all my theories. No matter.

It's always been that way since the dawn of civilization. Whenever something revolutionary is proposed, society is loathe to accept it. Picasso dealt with it, and eventually won. Einstein grappled with it and came out on top. So did thousands of others throughout history. I'm not putting myself in their class, but regardless, they give me inspiration.

The Warrior Diet is unlike any other modern diet plan. Every other modern eating plan is based on restraint. You count calories; you're careful about fat intake; you avoid carbohydrates. They tell you not to overeat or undereat. Well, I'm here to tell you that it doesn't have to be that way. The Warrior Diet is simple, effective, and ultimately, instinctual. It involves using the body's innate ability to burn fat and build muscle through the release of natural hormones and other growth factors. It doesn't involve any drugs. And it breaks all the rules. But that's what warriors do—they break the rules and shallow-minded restrictions placed on them by society.

Given that this mode of eating is so different from anything you've probably considered, I feel it necessary to offer some background before you learn the simple facts behind the Warrior Diet. After all, to accept anything merely on faith would be patently "un-warrior-like."

Ancient Warriors versus Modern Man

About one hundred thousand years ago, modern man reached his current state of evolution. At that point, his body, his genes, and his instincts pretty much reached their peak. The main thing that's really changed since then is how we now live—in a much more crowded, civilized world. Initially, we had to live by our instincts.

Now, they've been all but choked out of us. There's a reason, of course: following one's natural instincts is often dangerous to society. You can't very well let people go around doing every and anything they please.

In other words, in order to control people you have to control their most primitive instincts or desires.

Still, there are those who break rules. They are the true romantics of the world. They are the spiritual warriors and their actions often change the way we all live. Children start out as such romantics, but this instinct is usually beaten out of them by the time they reach adulthood. Consequently, there are very few modern warriors.

Thousands of years ago, these warriors were common. They lived entirely by instincts. In fact, whole societies were made up of warriors. They spent their days defending their lives and their families' lives. They moved from place to place, never stopping long enough to settle down. Generally, they only sat down to eat one meal a day, and that was always at night after the battles had been fought. Consequently, their bodies were lean and hard, and their instincts were honed to perfection.

You can even see these body types illustrated in ancient art. If you take a look at examples of Minoan art, the people depicted are lean, muscular, and heroic-looking. So, too, were the ancient Greeks and Romans. They were nomadic, eating one meal a day—mostly seasonal fresh food, meats, fish, legumes and whole grains, olive oil, and wine. However, if you look a little farther south to Egypt, long-revered for their magnificent civilization, you see something altogether different. Much of their art depicts a people very soft, almost feminine. The difference? They weren't nomads; they instead settled down and farmed the land. They had fewer battles to fight. They were a "rich" society, and consequently, many lived an aristocratic life, eating many meals throughout the day, much of which consisted of refined wheat and other grains, breads, and cakes.

The early Roman and Greek art reflected a warrior race. Soon after, though, decadence set in and they began living much the same way as modern man: with frequent meals, a sedentary life, and dulled instincts. Predictably they began to look like modern man and suffer the same ailments. (Until Nero, there wasn't one emperor who was obese.)

Clearly, the dietary habits of civilized modern man are very, very different from those of the ancient warrior. Civilized man lives largely off refined grains; eats often; and is reluctant to engage in intense physical pursuits. Contrast that with the warrior who consumed fresh, seasonal, and fermented food; ate sparingly during the day but filled himself up at night; and toiled during the day. Civilized man has grown fat and much of his unused muscle has atrophied. He lives by the clock, eating at predetermined times. The warrior, however, remained lean, hard, and muscular, living off his instincts and eating when necessary or when the workday was done.

One Meal A Day

By now, you've probably gotten an inkling of what kind of eating plan I've practiced for years and the one that's the subject of this book. The gist of the Warrior Diet is to eat a meal only once a day, preferably at night, and without any restriction of calories or macronutrient content.

It involves retraining the body (and the mind). If you try it for a few weeks, I maintain that your hunger will diminish during the day. And, when you eat at night, you'll know exactly what to eat and how much to eat. Your body may, in fact, tell you to eat a considerable amount—no matter, listen to it. During the day you'll likely want to nibble on things. This is okay, as long as your snack consists of fresh vegetables, fruits, and a little protein if desired, and doesn't include carbohydrates like breads or grains.

Yes, this runs against current theory. Yes, it runs against modern-day common sense. But there's a body of science to support it. We already know that exercising on an empty stomach stimulates more weight loss than if we had eaten beforehand. This diet guarantees you several hours a day of fat-burning hormones percolating through your body.

Long periods of undereating increases protein efficiency. If you refrain from eating large amounts of protein at arbitrary times, your body will become more efficient at recycling proteins, so when you do eat protein, it'll be utilized much more efficiently. Not eating for long periods also improves insulin sensitivity, so when you do eat, your blood sugar doesn't fluctuate wildly and your body won't store the carbohydrate calories as fat.

The list of potential benefits is staggering. Taking in certain types of protein on an empty stomach can increase testosterone levels and growth hormone levels, and you can't do that on a full stomach. Long periods of fasting also allow certain beneficial amino acids to act favorably on the brain. How many conventional diets do that?

Naysayers might argue that the body needs large reserves of glycogen to compete in athletic events. This may be true, but the Warrior Diet trains the body to stretch glycogen reserves so that athletic endurance doesn't become a problem. Others might point out that this type of diet may induce the production of the catabolic hormone cortisol, which may have negative effects on muscle growth and fat deposition. Ordinarily, yes, but this diet is not about water fasting. By ingesting the right nutrients during the Undereating Phase you will be able to block the cortisol effect.

Just to make sure we're on the same page, let's recap the essentials of the Warrior Diet. The main "trick" is to retrain your body; teach it to become more instinctive. You can do this by avoiding most foods during the day, although I do recommend that you eat vegetables and fruits (mainly as freshly squeezed juices). It's also okay to have a little protein during the day, such as eggs, lean fish, cheese, yogurt, or, preferably, undenatured whey. As you get used to eating this way, your cravings should disappear. And once you're done "fighting the battles" of the day, you can eat as much protein, vegetables, and carbs as you want—even if it means eating the equivalent of three meals in one seating.

The Warrior Diet Advantage

Make no mistake about it. This is not a three-week program or "get in shape for summer" plan. It is a lifestyle. As you continue to do it, hunger pangs during the day will likely disappear. Simultaneously, you'll find yourself getting leaner and more muscular. Furthermore, your thoughts should become clearer and more focused. You will, in short, become a warrior.

Remember, genetically we humans are hunter/collectors, as are predators in the forest. Wild animals, which practice "free feeding," stay lean and athletic, but when you put them in captivity they begin to eat like most modern human beings—nonstop. Their natural instincts wane and so they eat and eat, and eventually die.

Most people habitually eat between three to six small meals per day. Unfortunately, many are not satisfied with these small meals. Additionally, eating meals during the day leaves many people feeling sluggish and exhausted due to uncontrolled hormonal and neurotransmitter changes. On the other hand, when you practice the Warrior Diet, you can manipulate your hormones and neurotransmitters to work for you. In other words, instead of the hormones controlling the diet, your diet will control your hormones.

Although it may seem difficult to accept at first, the Warrior Diet allows you an incredible sense of freedom. Once your natural instincts kick in, you'll want to eat only one large meal per day, at night. You'll fully enjoy it and will get even more satisfaction knowing that you can eat to your heart's content. I believe that every time you fulfill an instinct there's a feeling of intense pleasure, a kind of high. We get this feeling from food, sex, and even after completing a workout. Could it be that the drive to exercise intensely is part of the "Warrior Instinct," and that people are drawn to bodybuilding or other sports because we're so deprived of this instinct in our modern lives?

I think so. It's all part of being a warrior.

"Warrior"—A New Definition

When I refer to the term "warrior," it is to an instinct that is deep within us all and which can be triggered by practicing the Warrior Diet.

The "Stubborn Fat" Syndrome

"Stubborn fat" is a major problem for many people today. Those who suffer from this "Stubborn Fat Syndrome" know that it's almost impossible to get rid of it. And they realize that even when they lose some body fat through diet and exercise, the fat they lose is not the stubborn fat. That's why it's called stubborn fat. This stubborn fat usually remains around the belly or chest area, making men look soft. On women, it usually hits their hips, butt, and thighs.

I'm not aware of any diet that seriously addresses this problem. It isn't a simple issue. One needs to understand what stubborn fat is, what the reasons are for having it, how to avoid it, why it's so hard to burn if you have it, and, most importantly, how to remove it. In Chapter 5 I explain how to deal with this syndrome. It's all part of the Warrior Diet.

Some Practical Advice

The Warrior Diet is simple and practical. However, since this book is full of information and ideas, it may seem a bit overwhelming at first. While I feel it is essential to ultimately read the whole book to fully understand all the concepts behind the Warrior Diet, you don't need to read it in its entirety before starting to practice it!

For those who want to begin the Warrior Diet without first breaking their teeth on all that's included, here is my advice:

Read the introduction to each chapter (as well as my preface and introduction at the beginning of the book). This will give you a clear indication of what it's about.

Once you understand the goals and follow the principles of the diet you'll be able to start practicing it. I believe that shortly after you begin the Warrior Diet you'll naturally be driven to learn more and more details because the effects of it may change your life. So, breaking the ice will, in time, come easily.

The goals and principles of the two main phases of the diet, Undereating and Overeating, are at the beginning of their respective chapters. "Warrior Meals and Recipes" offers some great meals and recipes to prepare, and the "Warrior Nutritional Supplements" suggests some nutritional supplements you may want to take. Reading these chapters should make it easy for anyone to follow the Warrior Diet.

To sum up, I think any diet is practical if:

First:	**One understands the goals**
Second:	**One understands the principles**
Third:	**One has access to the right nutritional foods**
Fourth:	**One is able to follow it on a daily basis, enjoy it, and feel satisfied.**

It's all here!

THE WARRIOR DIET PRINCIPLE:

- The Warrior Diet is based on a daily cycle of undereating and overeating.

THE WARRIOR DIET GOALS:

1. Trigger the Warrior Instinct
2. Burn Fat
3. Build Muscles
4. Accelerate Metabolism
5. Boost Neurotransmitters
6. Detoxify
7. Slow the Aging Process
8. Attain a Sense of Freedom
9. Reach Satisfaction
10. Live Instinctively

WARRIOR DIET

CHAPTER ONE
THE WARRIOR
INSTINCT

There's a primal instinct deep inside you that may be triggered in (what I call) moments of truth. This instinct spontaneously guides how you act, react, compete, fight, or hunt when faced with different situations or events that require an action or reaction in order to survive—without compromising your freedom to be what and who you really are. I call this the "Warrior Instinct."

The question remains: What really triggers this "Warrior Instinct?" My answer, all through this book, is the Warrior Diet. Once you get on the "Warrior Cycle" you trigger this awesome instinct.

This chapter is devoted to all aspects of this primal force, including how the "Warrior Instinct" manifests itself through three other human instincts:

- The Instinct to Survive and Multiply
- The Hunter/Predator Instinct
- The Scavenger Instinct

I believe strongly that the "Warrior Instinct," the Instinct to Survive and Multiply, the Hunter/Predator Instinct, and the Scavenger Instinct are all related and come from the same source, and that they're all eventually connected to the Warrior Diet. Another instinct, that I call the Romantic Instinct, is discussed in Chapter 8, the "Warrior Idea," as I believe it is also a manifestation of the "Warrior Instinct."

There's much more to all this, so please keep reading.

The Instinct to Survive and Multiply

Two basic instincts guide us throughout our lives, and the "Warrior Instinct" controls and allows them to manifest. The Instinct to Survive ensures that we keep ourselves alive, by protecting ourselves, and hunting for food. Human beings are hunter/collectors, and the fact that we are hunters by nature places us in the category of predators. This Hunter Instinct is part of our survival instinct, and with it comes the aggression to do two things: protect our lives and kill, if necessary.

The Instinct to Multiply gives the human species, like any other species, the desire to engage in sex and produce offspring in order to keep the race alive and well, and ensure future generations.

There is also competition between males and females, respectively, to select the best mate. This involves the "Warrior Instinct." When triggered, you try to demonstrate your superiority, uniqueness, continually improving yourself to be able to compete for the best mate so that you can produce the best possible offspring to carry your genes. Throughout history, this has been the case with both humans and animals. Humans, civilized creatures that we are, control and repress these primal instincts. I believe, however, that people cannot inhibit them completely, since they remain deep in the subconscious—like a volcano about to explode.

By now you're probably asking yourself why I'm talking about this in a diet book. It all ties together and relates to the Warrior Diet. It will all make sense soon.

The Hunter Instinct

Hunters have always intrigued and fascinated me. The Warrior Diet mimics the way classical hunters cycled between phases of undereating (controlled fasting) and overeating (compensation).

We all know that in the past humans had to hunt for food in order to survive. Hunting gave the hunter an adrenal rush, as it should, and a whole culture of ritualistic behavior. For instance, when stalking large animals, hunters usually went in groups. At the end of the day, when the mission was accomplished, there was a ritual of compensation—cutting the meat, creating a feast, compensating all who took part, including the animals that helped, like the dogs (British hunters dipped a piece of bread in the quarry's blood and gave this to the dogs as a reward for their hard work).

So, the day consisted of two periods, hunting and compensation. Most of the day was devoted to the hardship of hunting and then preparing the meal, and at the end of the day all were compensated. The entire cycle is important. Neither can be missing.

Today, when we no longer need to hunt for food and the "Warrior Instinct" is inhibited by its aggressive, antiestablishment connotations, many people still find ways to feel and experience their "Warrior Instinct." This is evident in most competitive sports, which closely mimic the experience of hunting. Another example is how some sport hunters today don't use guns, choosing instead to use traditional methods like a bow and arrow, or by stabbing the animal. This may sound primitive or extreme to most, but it appeals to and satisfies a primal instinct.

Here is another example of hunting that is closely related to the Warrior Diet:

Falconry

In the ancient tradition of "Falconry," falcons are taught how to hunt. They learn to fly above their trainers, who follow on horseback until the falcon catches a bird and drops him down.

Falconry is still practiced in the British Islands, other parts of Europe, and especially in the Mediterranean and the Middle East. Hunters in these regions of the world adore falcons and think of them as "the ultimate bird." Some even compare them to humans in a positive way (or at least with a positive aspect). The eagle, which is within the same family of hunting birds, has been and is today a symbol of many nations.

The methods used to train falcons are worth noting. In order to keep this bird in captivity without losing its Predator Instinct, trainers created what I call a "cycling diet": the falcon is deprived of food for most of the day and is then fed fresh meat, just enough to give them the taste of blood. This deprivation of food keeps their "Warrior Instinct" alive, and their Hunter Instinct sharp. The cycling diet keeps them strong and aggressive enough to catch their prey.

Cycling the falcons' diet with fasting and then feeding mimics the way that they eat in the wild, hunting whenever hungry and fasting when not. If you feed a falcon even a little bit too much, he loses the desire to hunt, loses his vitality, and loses his alertness. A hungry falcon is in his best shape. So, they are trained to hunt on an empty stomach.

The other key element in training falcons consists of playing with them, using a stick with fresh, raw meat on top, which the trainers move in the air, allowing the falcons to fly and catch it. The distance of the play is gradually increased. It is like a "virtual-reality" game of hunting birds in flight. And this is how the bird exercises.

I feel empathy toward this beautiful bird, and believe that falconry not just symbolizes but also parallels how human beings are supposed to live. Yet most of us no longer live in the woods, hunting and gathering food. Instead we live in crowded urban environments, in the suburbs, or even rural communities, with busy schedules, working in offices, carrying briefcases, with around the clock routines, far from a purely natural lifestyle. And most of our primal instincts are crushed on a daily basis. We are basically living in a very unwarrior-like, almost captive, situation.

But, like a falcon, if you want to, you can turn this virtual reality into reality and trigger your "Warrior Instinct"—without going to war, needing to kill anything, or even changing jobs. All you must do is keep a cycling diet, which is built on the essence of extremes: undereating, which I call controlled fasting; and feeding/overeating, which I call compensation. When following a cycling diet you'll get both feelings — hunger and satiety, deprivation and compensation. Another key component of the Warrior Diet is exercise. This will be discussed in the "Warrior Workout" chapter.

As mentioned before, I believe that human beings by nature are hunters, and that many successful people have similarities to predators. Therefore, it's interesting to look at what happens to wild animals when they are caged for an extended period of time.

Predators in the Wild vs. Predators in Captivity

A lot can be learned when looking at the differences in behavior between predators in the wild, and those that live in captivity.

When a wild predator, such as a lion, hunts and eats its kill, it eats in safety and only to the point of satiety. Then it leaves and the surviving prey know that the lion is no longer a threat, at least for the time being, simply because lions don't hunt when they are not hungry. They become peaceful. They lie on their back, enjoy the sun, and sleep. However, when you put predators in a cage they often eat and eat (bingeing) and usually don't stop until they get sick. They will eventually die if their captors don't control their feedings.

I give this example because I feel there are also some similarities between human beings and caged predators. Too many of us, for instance, eat several meals throughout the day and evening, sometimes even when full—without reaching satisfaction. If this continues unabated, it'll likely cause sickness.

I've come to the conclusion there are two main reasons why people eat like this:

1. They feel liked caged predators.
2. They've lost their instinct.

Sadly, most of us are not aware that our eating habits, and what we consume, are major reasons why we become sick, overweight, age prematurely, etc., or of the fact that we have the power to choose whether to live like a free predator or a caged animal.

Here's the opposite spectrum, what I call the Scavenger Instinct.

The Scavenger Instinct

There are several distinct differences between hunters and scavengers. Hunters/predators work in order to get their food. They make a selection. They know exactly what they are after. Wild cats do not hunt cucumbers. They hunt rabbits and deer. They eat only when hungry. They have a sense of priority—and a sense of time. This is very important. When a hunter/predator is about to eat his kill, he may be in danger if there are other animals around. If this is the case, he'll tear it apart, taking the best chunk and run with it to a safe place to eat. When necessary, he'll fight for the first bite. Hunters/ predators like to eat when it's safe and they can relax. Some animals, like wolves or mountain lions, will take the food, bury it, and come back at night (when it's safe) to dig it out. Their instincts are sharp.

The scavenger is exactly the opposite. While hunters work hard to get their food, scavengers don't. They pick up leftovers. While hunters have a sense of priority and know exactly what they need, scavengers have no clear sense of priority. While hunters will make a selection, choosing their food, scavengers eat whatever is available. While hunters eat only when hungry, scavengers eat all the time. While hunters eat warm, fresh, live food, the scavenger often eats cold, dead food. While hunters like to eat when it's safe so they can relax, scavengers eat "on the go." These comparisons might make you wonder what kind of person you are. Are you a hunter/predator or a scavenger? Be honest with yourself. Which do you want to be?

Can You Be a Hunter Without Hunting?

You may ask, "Are we all forced scavengers?" The answer is mostly yes. "Are there really hunters any more?" My answer is that even though most of us no longer hunt in a traditional sense for our food, the Hunter Instinct is within us all—and you can easily switch it on.

"Can you be a hunter if you choose your food but purchase it in advance?"

Good question.

With awareness, by choosing your own food you're already working for it and making priorities. Once you reach the peak—by designing your meals, cooking your food, and understanding what tastes do for you—you are living like a hunter. You understand what you want, set your priorities, acquire your food and, as necessary, prepare it, all of which requires effort. You sit down for your meals and relax. Then when you eat you're satisfied and you don't need to eat more. People who shop in health food stores, even if they don't understand exactly what they're doing, are already a big step ahead because they at least have awareness and are making priorities and choices. The scavenger, by contrast, is like an idiot. An idiot is someone who doesn't think about what he's doing. A scavenger will pick up any food, not knowing its nutritional value or where it came from, nor care if it's fresh, and eat it—just for the sake of eating.

Thousands of years ago, hunting and eating fresh kill were a necessary part of life in order to survive. The later development of raising animals on farms, which dominates the way we eat meat today, crushes the "traditional" Hunter Instinct.

Today, the vast majority of these farm-raised animals are given hormones in order to gain weight rapidly. For the meat industry, time is money and, yes, we are the victims. We are forced to scavenge what's available in the supermarket, most of which is drugged, loaded with chemicals, and is therefore contaminated meat. I believe that the mainstream food industry has been largely responsible for turning people into scavengers by supplying and heavily promoting overly processed foods with aggressive tastes, lacking freshness and nutritional value.

You can mimic your Hunter Instinct by refusing to buy meat filled with hormones or other drugs, or fed rendered feed. Instead, seek out and buy organic meat that comes from animals that were treated in a humane way, fed freely on grass and grain, and were not injected with estrogen, growth hormones, or antibiotics. It might be more expensive, but your body will be healthier and your life more expansive. Don't ever think otherwise.

Hopefully I've put this all in perspective and you're now in touch with (or at least aware of) this deep primal instinct within you, and within all of us—the "Warrior Instinct."

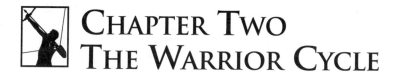

CHAPTER TWO
THE WARRIOR CYCLE

The Human Cycle

We naturally do everything in cycles: eat, drink, go to the bathroom, sleep and awaken. Our body is cycling nonstop, things going in, things going out. When one of these processes is blocked you become imbalanced, sick, and you may eventually die if it's not corrected. Our brains react to the cycle of day and night, especially through the pineal gland and the pituitary, which secrete hormones. I believe awareness of these cycles is instinctual, that everyone has his or her own cycle, and each time you break it, you're going to feel it.

Some even believe that life itself is a cycle. That once you die your soul is going to recycle to another life and that the people you knew in this life were part of your former life and will be again in your next. Whether this is true is beside the point. I'll try to illustrate in this chapter that there is indeed a human cycle and that it's built on extremes.

The Warrior Cycle

The Warrior Diet is built on the principle of cycling between periods of undereating and overeating, based on an instinct deep within us to undereat and overeat. The combination of undereating and overeating is not endorsed by mainstream diets; they are against this principle. Yet I truly believe the "Warrior Cycle" is the only biological cycle that we are built for, and are naturally meant to live by. Any other method compromises our true nature.

The different aspects of the "Warrior Cycle" are:

• The Energetic Cycle
• The Cycle of Materialism and Dematerialism
• The Healing Process of the Cycle
• Finding the Right Cycle for Optimum Results—Timing

Each is discussed here, as well as how they relate to the Warrior Diet.

The Energetic Cycle

When Einstein introduced his theory of relativity, it was just that: a theory. It wasn't proven until years later. When asked what he'd say if his theory was not correct, he replied that he would feel sorry for God almighty if such a beautiful theory didn't work.

Today we know that there is unity between matter and energy, that material can turn into energy, and energy can turn into material. The exact connection between quantum mechanics and macro-mechanics is still not known, but it is acknowledged that there's a connection. Whether our spirit and soul are pure energy, and our body pure material is not known. One thing for sure is that without energy we are dead, so we are not just material. Even though we think of the world in a materialistic way, we actually sense it through energy. All our cells are built to survive and function through quantum mechanic principles.

Moreover, people throughout the world believe that material can move into spirit and spirit into material. They believe that when we die all we lose is the material, our body, but the spirit will go on. They believe in past lives, future lives, and in cycles. No matter what your belief, it's clear that the role energy plays in the universe is quite predominant.

Here is how this is connected to the Warrior Diet:

The Cycle of Materialism and Dematerialism

What happens in your body during the "Undereating Phase" of the Warrior Diet is what I call dematerialization, meaning that you remove/eliminate more material than you put inside. Basically, burned material turns into energy. Once you learn how to undereat and begin to practice it, you'll find that you have more energy, are more productive, more creative, more ambitious, and hungrier for life. This expanded "hunger for life" occurs when your body and mind are in a state of turning material into energy.

On the other hand, when feeding is frequent (between three and six meals) throughout the day, the opposite may occur and many people may gain weight. Why? When material (food) is continually added to the body, much of our energy must be devoted to digesting and eliminating it. The body often doesn't produce enough energy to eliminate it all. When this is the case, one becomes "overmaterialized" and the body is overwhelmed. Lethargy, exhaustion, and bloating are the result. Additionally, the excess material is deposited as body fat, and stored as toxins. On top of all this, some undigested material eventually reaches the bloodstream, which can trigger allergic reactions and may lead to full-blown diseases.

The Healing Process of the Cycle

A most important aspect of the Warrior Diet is the healing process. What does this really mean? And, how do you prevent illnesses and keep your mind and body healthy? To me, you can't truly understand what health and healing are unless you understand what illness is and are able to recognize its symptoms. Philosophically speaking, perhaps illness was sent to us in order to understand how to be healthy.

Just as a warrior must anticipate his enemy's behavior and reactions and understand the dangers, and just as a hunter must know the behavior patterns of animals that he hunts, in order for us to heal, achieve, and maintain a state of mental and physical health, we must be in touch with our body and be aware of the symptoms of illness.

Our ability to heal, and the healing process itself, should never be taken for granted. Vanity often keeps us from accepting that we'll all inevitably face cycles of being weaker and stronger, sicker and healthier. This isn't just a slogan. Look at it like this: When you want to build muscle and get strong, you first have to break the fiber. Only then is the body tricked into a healing process to rebuild the tissue. This is similar to how the immune system is built after being exposed to colds, viruses, infections, etc.

Acupuncture heals by inserting tiny needles into certain places on the body that are energy sensors and pathways. The tiny incisions that penetrate the skin create a healing process.

Similarly, every time you undereat by following the Warrior Diet rules, your body has the potential to heal. Undereating (controlled fasting) triggers healing in two major ways: first, you will have more energy available since it's not being used for digestion, and second because of the detoxification process that occurs during this phase. Then when you eat a meal it completes the compensation process and gives you a sense of freedom and satisfaction. On the other hand, when you eat several meals throughout the day, you don't give your body a chance to go through the processes of detoxification and healing or deprivation and satisfaction.

The "Undereating Phase" of the Warrior Diet basically empowers you both physically and mentally to finish the day with compensation.

Every day has a happy end. So, you go through two extreme periods: first the "Undereating Phase," when you are very alert, energetic, active, productive, "hungry for life," and then the "Overeating Phase," when you cool out, calm down and are fully compensated.

All in the Timing: Finding Your Cycle

It's crucial to determine the right cycle, and to find harmony when moving between undereating and overeating. The "Undereating Phase" should not last longer than 16—18 hours. If it goes beyond this, the body usually starts to draw from its lean tissues because the available material used for energy has been completely depleted. Your potential energy will decrease when fasting or undereating for too long. This is self-destructive and dangerous to your health. You'll become weak, and possibly anorexic. That's why it's the art of controlled fasting that keeps your metabolism high. Once you find the right cycle, all will be balanced and you'll see your body become stronger, leaner, cleaner, and healthier.

Moreover, an integral component of the "Undereating Phase" of the Warrior Diet is that it should be done while you are awake. This is the time to produce energy out of matter. Because your body is not being burdened with breaking down and digesting food, you'll have lots of energy to think, create, produce, be ambitious, and, figuratively, to "go for the hunt." This is also when the sympathetic nervous system—the system that controls the "fight or flight" instincts—is dominant.

The sleeping hours are when your body needs to rejuvenate, recuperate, and rebuild. This is the time when the parasympathetic nervous system—the system that controls digestion and elimination—is dominant. Your body will serve you better if you follow the "Warrior Cycle."

Moreover, an integral component of the "Undereating Phase" of the Warrior Diet is that it should be done while you are awake. This is the time to produce energy out of matter. Because your body is not being burdened with breaking down and digesting food, you'll have lots of energy to think, create, produce, be ambitious, and, figuratively, to "go for the hunt." This is also when the sympathetic nervous system—the system that controls the "fight or flight" instincts—is dominant.

CHAPTER THREE
THE UNDEREATING
PHASE

"Yond Cassius has a lean and hungry look;
He thinks too much: such men are dangerous."
—William Shakespeare, *Julius Caesar,* Act I, Scene 2

For most people, undereating means not eating enough. Actually, what it really means for you is not eating as much as you used to eat during the day. This may sound so simple, and maybe it is, but there is much more to it.

In this chapter I explain what controlled fasting is, why it's so essential for optimizing your energy and performance, and how exactly to put it into practice. The key to maintaining the Warrior Diet is related to this phase, so please stay with me.

The Undereating Phase is the first part of the Warrior Cycle, lasting most of the day. It's the time that requires more energy—physical, mental, and spiritual. This is when you are working, learning, creating, competing, doing physical activities, and often struggling through the hardships of your day. The Undereating Phase, as you'll see, nourishes your brain while accelerating fat burning hour-by-hour, on a daily basis.

The first part of this chapter covers the different aspects of controlled fasting, including:

• What Happens to Your Body During Fasting
• The Fear of Hunger
• How to Deal with Hunger
• What Fasting is Exactly on The Warrior Diet

Part Two of this chapter covers the subject of daily detoxification, which is a major goal of the Warrior Diet. I also explain that by manipulating your hormones you naturally guarantee hours of fat burning, day by day.

In Part Three you'll find some practical information on the adaptation period, which ought to help your body adapt to the Warrior Diet.

Once you go over all of this, hopefully you'll find that it makes sense. By practicing the Undereating Phase you should discover that you'll become leaner, more vigorous—and, I believe, more focused.

Before you begin to practice this phase, it's necessary to understand two fundamentals:

1. The Undereating Principle
2. The Undereating Goals

The Undereating Principle

The Undereating Phase is built on the principle of controlled fasting. It lasts for 16–18 hours after your last meal, including time you are asleep. During this phase, you can consume "live": fresh, raw fruits and vegetables, and some protein.

The Undereating Goals

- Burn fat
- Detoxify and cleanse
- Manipulate your hormones to reach maximum metabolic efficiency

Part One
Controlled Fasting

The Undereating Phase can be followed by not eating anything. Some people like water fasts, while others prefer to drink coffee or tea and water only. This is okay if it's what you like to do. However, these are extreme methods that won't appeal to most people. Moreover, I believe that the best way of going through the Undereating Phase is by following a controlled fast, not a water fast. Controlled fasting is easier to follow and it accelerates detoxification and overall well-being.

To practice the Undereating Phase, it's very important to understand what controlled fasting and hunger are— as well as their different aspects. This is essential reading for following the Warrior Diet.

What happens to your body during controlled fasting:

- Detoxification takes effect (a cleansing)
- The body's enzyme pool is reloaded (which accelerates fat burning and toning, as well as creating an anti-aging effect)
- Insulin drops and is stabilized (efficient metabolism of carbs and fats)
- Glucagon increases (a fat-burning hormone)
- The GH increases (tissue repair and fat burning)

Here is briefly what happens:

When you fast, insulin drops and the hormone glucagon increases, to ensure a steady supply of energy to the body. When glucagon dominates, most of the body's energy is derived from glycogen reserves and fat stores. Also, the drop in insulin allows the growth hormone (GH) to peak. Elevation of GH helps the body to rejuvenate, repair tissues, and burn fat. A natural elevation of GH on a daily basis, I believe, should help slow the aging process. Unfortunately, GH is deactivated under acidic environments. Most people suffer from overacidity as a result of over-consumption of acid-forming foods, a lack of digestive enzymes, mineral deficiencies, and physical or mental stress.

The advantage of controlled fasting is the alkalizing effect that "live" fruits and vegetables, and their juices, have on the body, which is further pronounced by taking ionized mineral supplements. Ionized minerals are the most potent biologically active minerals, and they provide an instant, alkalizing action. When GH is elevated in an alkalized body, it will reach its maximum metabolic efficiency.

Let's now look at the different aspects of hunger and fasting:

The Fear of Hunger

Many people today have an irrational—almost phobic—fear of going hungry. We live in a society that teaches us it isn't good to ever be hungry, and that hunger can even be dangerous. Of course, this is partly true since everyone needs to eat, and when you're hungry it triggers the *reactive* part of the survival instinct (which says "I must eat in order to survive"). But when you know how to manipulate hunger *correctly*, it will serve you in many positive ways. Hunger will trigger the *active* part of the survival instinct— that which makes you more alert, ambitious, competitive, and creative.

Throughout history, humans have had to contend with hunger, and not just because they were unable to afford food, or suffered from drought and famine. Learning to deal with hunger was also practiced intentionally, to make people tougher and stronger, to better handle life's hardships.

The historical correlation between hunger and freedom is quite evident. During the period when the Bible was written, and later, during the Roman Empire, hunger and fasting were considered an integral part of life for free people, warriors, and those who wandered.

Slaves, on the other hand, were fed frequently throughout the day. The Israelite slaves' first complaint after escaping from slavery in Egypt, was of hunger, and they wandered in the desert for forty years, adapting, and eventually becoming a free nation. Only the second generation of these slaves reached the Promised Land.

I firmly believe that hunger triggers the Warrior Instinct and if it's under control will give you a "sense of freedom." I also believe that frequently feeding—from a fear of hunger—may, to put it strongly, create a "slave mentality," because when fed continually, people tend to become more lethargic, lazy, and submissive—and thus easily controlled.

How to Deal with Hunger

First, you should know that when you control hunger, it isn't going to harm you, so you shouldn't be afraid of it. During a controlled fast the hunger sensations usually don't last more than a few minutes, after which there is an adaptation in the body to the stress of hunger—and the feeling should dissipate.

The second thing you should understand is that hunger is a sign of vitality and health.

Third, when you do feel hungry, go ahead and have a piece of fruit, or a freshly squeezed vegetable or fruit juice. If you feel you also need some protein, eat a small portion, with small amounts of raw green vegetables. (Go to Chapter 4, "What To Consume During The Undereating Phase" for more on this). Take advantage of your energy and alertness. In time you should adapt, find that you no longer suffer during this phase, and will enjoy a general feeling of well-being.

Excruciating hunger is, however, a different story. When your body is chronically depleted of essential nutrients, such as when you fast for more than 18 hours or are starving, you may feel extreme hunger that's almost like a pain. You should listen to your body and eat. It's always good to break a fast with fresh vegetable or fruit juice.

What Fasting Means

Fasting means different things to different people. Islamic people, for instance, fast during Ramadan. To them, it means not eating during the day, and eating only at night. Roman Catholics fast during Lent, avoiding meat. Orthodox Jews completely avoid all foods and drink, including water, during the Yom Kippur fast. In the past, Jewish spiritual leaders went on a mono diet. They lived solely on figs and carob fruits. In the East, spiritual leaders used to practice water fasting, some for short periods of time, and others for a couple of months. During the Roman Empire, Romans fasted, eating only peas. Today fasting is becoming ever more popular, especially among people who want to lose weight, or do a natural cleansing.

What Fasting Means
on the Warrior Diet

On the Warrior Diet, the principle of fasting is based on not eating a full meal during the day. Since the Undereating Phase lasts for most of the day, you can consume certain "live" foods and should drink a lot of water. Naturally stimulating beverages, such as coffee and tea, are allowed, and a few nutritional supplements are suggested. You must, however, minimize the amount of food to mostly live (raw) food, in the form of fruit and veggies and their natural juices—and a small portion of protein if needed. This keeps your digestive system untaxed and continues to manipulate your hormones to the optimum balance. Choose your food and beverages carefully, to accelerate detoxification. Processed carbs and sugars should be avoided during this phase, so as not to boost your insulin levels.

Fasting versus Starvation

There is a *significant difference* between fasting and starvation. Fasting is the art of manipulating the metabolic system; it is controlled, and for a limited time. When you reach this peak time period, and then eat a large meal, your metabolism will be boosted higher than it was before. Conversely, with starvation, the fasting is not controlled. Your metabolism will slow down and you will start to "cannibalize" your muscles and lean tissues. Starvation slows the metabolism and, if done chronically, may even lead to death.

The Spiritual Side of Fasting

Many different religions, including Hinduism, Islam, Christianity, and Judaism, consider adult fasting a way to reach a deeper spiritual level. There also seems to be a natural connection between controlled fasting and becoming less materialistic. During a fast, material in the body is turned into energy, and I believe this alone makes one less materialistic and more spiritual.

The Hunger For Life

As I've mentioned before, during this time you're moving from the material world into an energetic, creative one. On the scientific side, the hormonal balance is different when you fast than it is after you eat. After you eat a full meal, including carbs, the insulin system is dominant. Insulin deposits material (both protein and fat) into your tissues.

On the other hand, during a controlled fast, the glucagon system takes over from the insulin system and removes material from your body, turning fat into energy. So, during the controlled fasting time, you move away from what I call a "materialistic metabolism" to an "energetic metabolism." Once you adapt to controlled fasting, you should experience what I call a "hunger for life." Your Warrior Instinct will kick in and you'll become sharper, more alert, more energetic, and more adventurous.

A Few Words on Fasting to Heal

Children fast instinctively when they are sick; so do animals. And for many years, when people wanted to heal, they took a fast.

Overall mind-body energy is increased with fasting. This healing force throws off accumulated toxins, clears dead cells, and rebalances and rejuvenates the body. Paul Bragg, author of *The Miracle of Fasting*, states: "The greatest discovery by modern man is the power to rejuvenate himself physically, mentally, and spiritually with rational fasting."

Some researchers believe that cancerous cells die in alkaline environments. They theorize that manipulating the correct pH through fasting can accelerate the destruction of sick cells and tumors, which thrive in acid environments. There is also much research on enzyme healing, alleviation from depression, as well as natural toxin elimination. World-renowned fasting expert Dr. Buchinger describes fasting as "the burning of rubbish." I'll touch on these subjects in more detail soon.

Part Two

Daily Detoxification (Elimination of Toxins; Burning Fat; Anti-Aging)

The accumulation of material in your body, especially undigested foods and toxins, makes you sick. To begin with, avoiding toxins is very important, but it's at least as important to give your body the chance to detoxify itself. This is key for your health. When you follow traditional diets, eating three to six meals a day, your body doesn't have enough time to get rid of all the material. Detoxification, in my opinion, is the most important thing you can do to live longer and have a healthier, attractive body.

When you detoxify, a cleansing takes effect. There is a natural wisdom of the body to remove toxins. Unfortunately, when too many toxins are ingested, the overwhelmed body can't get rid of them all. And when toxins remain, building up over time, it leads to ever-greater health risks. Since we consume, breathe, and absorb so many contaminants and pollutants through our skin, lungs, and gastrointestinal tract every day, I firmly believe it's important to detoxify on a daily basis.

> The Warrior Diet is the only diet I'm aware of that's based on daily detoxification—without, as I've said before, deprivation. There is no other diet that includes these two elements: detoxification, and then eating as much as you want.

We'll cover here the different aspects of daily detoxification, as well as three awesome properties of the Undereating Phase:

- Anti-Aging (Through Enzyme Loading)
- Fat Burning (Through Hormonal Manipulation)
- Killing Tumors and Cancerous Cells (Through Detoxification)

What is Detoxification?

Detoxification is literally the neutralizing, breaking down, and elimination of waste and toxins from the body. Every human organism and cell has what I call "anabolic and catabolic life cycles." The anabolic process deposits material, whether good or bad, protein, fat, or toxins, into the tissues. The catabolic process destroys and takes material away from the body, whether it's through burning fat, eliminating waste or removing toxins. *This cycle of depositing material and removing material should be done on a daily basis. If one of these processes does not happen properly, you will eventually get sick.*

Detoxification ensures the elimination of waste and removal of toxins. This is an essential part of the life cycle. Unfortunately, most people today do not eliminate enough. To be brutally honest, I would say that many people are in fact constipated and chronically loaded with toxins. And it's not just because they eat the wrong food. It's also because they don't give their bodies enough time to detoxify. Time is a very important factor in the Warrior Diet—indeed it is one of the factors that makes this diet so special and unique.

Elimination

Elimination is integral to detoxification. It's also a vital part of the daily human cycle, or the Warrior Cycle. It is believed that constipation and other elimination-related disorders are the main causes of most disease, as well as of premature aging. The Warrior Diet promotes a natural, healthy elimination cycle.

Destroying Sick Cells and Tumors

More and more research shows that fasting and detoxification helps attack and kill sick cells and tumors. Cancer cells thrive on sugar and acid environments. Daily fasting eliminates excess sugar from the cells, and the alkalizing effect of "live" fruits and veggies (and their juices) aids in rejuvenating healthy cells while helping to destroy sick cells. Enzyme loading accelerates the healing process. More on this is found in the next chapter under "Enzyme Loading."

Your immune system is naturally boosted during fasting and detoxification. When the immune system is intact, the body recognizes sick cells as "foreign invaders" and will try to destroy them. Daily detoxification and fasting are key to activate this immune response. In my opinion, fasting daily works like a natural chemotherapy and detoxifying daily is the best natural way to let the body defend itself. It takes time to detoxify, and the Warrior Diet gives your body this vital time through the Undereating Phase.

Detoxification and the Healing Process

Detoxification brings on a healing process. Most people that I know who have gone through this process have done so with no side effects. However, when the body is overburdened with toxins, it may sometimes produce temporary and uncomfortable symptoms as toxins are eliminated. For instance, you may get allergic reactions, like a runny nose or skin rashes, or experience flu-like symptoms. People don't usually realize that these symptoms are the body's way of naturally activating the immune cleanse itself by getting rid of toxins in any available way. Instead of letting nature do its job, many people today try to eliminate these symptoms by taking drugs. The mainstream pharmaceutical and medical communities compound this problem by advocating, promoting, and selling quick-fix medicines to mask the effects or reduce these symptoms, making a fortune in the process.

If, for instance, you have a fever and do not take a drug to relieve it, in most cases the fever will kill the bacteria or other pathogens, thus helping the body to detoxify and heal. Taking drugs cuts short this process, so your body may not have the chance to finish the healing cycle. It's important to realize that some unpleasant symptoms are normal, and you should try to overcome them without interference. (There are also natural ways to reduce them such as taking minerals, vitamins and antioxidants. We'll discuss these later.) The cleaner your body is, the fewer symptoms you will get. As noted, most people I know that have gone on the Warrior Diet did not face any unpleasant symptoms; in fact, quite the opposite. Most felt better and almost immediately experienced a greater increase in energy.

Manipulating Hormones and Neurotransmitters to Maximum Metabolic Efficiency

During the Undereating (controlled-fasting) Phase, growth hormone, insulin, glucagon, and cortisol (the stress hormone) are all manipulated naturally to optimum balance. You may ask why you want to manipulate these hormones. My answer: to reach a peak of metabolic efficiency, to burn fat, and to rejuvenate your body overall.

Manipulating your hormones has certain important benefits:

• Anti-aging: Elevation of growth hormone (GH) can help provide anti-aging effects.

• Burning Fat: When the hormones and enzymes that burn fat are working at an accelerated rate (through elevation of GH, glucagon, lipase, and the decline of the insulin hormone).

• Vigor: You will feel potent, powerful, and more positive (by opening the "brain barrier," boosting brain neurotransmitters through improved blood circulation, and blocking of cortisol).

When you know how to naturally manipulate your hormones and brain neurotransmitters, which are the best energy controllers in your body, you can reach your most energetic state.

Part Three
The Adaptation Period

Adapting to the Warrior Cycle is a necessary component of the Undereating Phase. During this time your body will get stronger and stronger. The adaptation period usually lasts for the first few weeks when beginning the Warrior Diet. Some people adapt immediately, but it normally takes between one to three weeks.

In the past, we humans (including children) adapted more easily to different situations because we were forced to face times of real hardship and pressure, like famines, and so had no choice.

With all changes in lifestyles, careers, etc., and in order to continue to grow stronger, adaptation is necessary. Adaptation relates to the Warrior Instinct (see Chapter One) because part of the Warrior Instinct involves taking chances.

Once you have adapted, you should feel great and full of energy during this phase— not to mention how exhilarated you'll feel once you've liberated yourself from old habits. And, you can look forward to true satiety because you will soon be eating as much as you want. The Overeating Phase is just around the corner.

If You Find It Difficult to Adapt

Some people find it difficult to jump right into the Warrior Diet all at once. If this is the case for you, I recommend that you begin to practice it gradually. Here are two suggestions:

1. Gradually increase the controlled-fasting time.

Start by undereating from morning until noon, and then add an hour or two per day. In a matter of a few weeks, you'll get used to it and will probably enjoy it. Remember, you're allowed to consume certain foods during the Undereating Phase. The Warrior Diet is not a water fast.

2. Gradually increase the days that you practice the Warrior Diet.

Start by practicing the Warrior Diet one or two days per week. Increase to three or four days the following week, then to five or six the week after that, and so on until you're fully adapted.

As I said, it's better for some people to ease in gradually, than to jump in cold turkey, so take your time with the adaptation period if this is the case for you.

Many of the people I know who have tried the Warrior Diet have said that they almost immediately experienced such tremendous improvement, both physically and mentally, that they felt confident they were on the right track and found it quite easy to change their eating habits.

Do what's good for you.

Chapter Four
What to Consume During the Undereating Phase

This chapter covers the different foods and nutritional supplements you can consume during the Undereating Phase. At the end of the chapter I offer my review of protein powders, for those who like to consume them during the day.

Detoxification and keeping insulin at a minimal level are of prime importance during the Undereating Phase.

"Living" Foods

It's most important to consume live (raw) foods on a daily basis during the Undereating Phase. Live foods contain vital nutrients, enzymes, vitamins, and minerals that aid in daily detoxification. The importance of live foods goes beyond the vitamins and minerals you get from them.

What Are "Living" Foods For The Undereating Phase?

"Living foods" are fresh, raw fruits and vegetables, as well as freshly squeezed fruit and vegetable juices. I mean really fresh fruits, really fresh vegetables, and really fresh juices, not those sold pre-made.

Advantages to Eating Living Foods

Living foods contain many vital live ingredients. They are the highest source of food enzymes, vitamins, minerals, and other phytonutrients in their most active state. They are critical for your health.

When you ingest raw fruits and veggies, or freshly squeezed veggie and fruit juices, you reload your body with living enzymes. And every time you reload your body with living enzymes, you optimize your body to:

1. Detoxify and create an antiaging effect.
2. Reduce inflammation, congestion, and pain.
3. Better digest the food that you will eat later during the Overeating Phase.
4. Replenish your body with nature's life forces.

Processed Foods Vs. Live-Food

Most processing—including many cooking methods, heat, acid-processing, and pasteurization—destroys the food's enzymes and probiotics (the friendly bacteria in your gastrointestinal system). Processing can denature protein and fats. However, special processing techniques, like controlled low-temperature, freeze-dried, or air-dried techniques, can preserve the vitality and integrity of living foods. You could say that the term "living food" is a relative matter. Fresh, raw foods are most alive, and from there it begins a downhill slide until food is technically dead. The processed-food industry does a wonderful job wrapping up and selling dead food in a way that makes it look alive and attractive. But, as a warrior, you should be able to tell the difference between what's alive and what's dead.

What to Drink

It's extremely important to drink a lot of fluids throughout the day, primarily water. Vegetable juices that are freshly prepared in a juicer are the best choice to complement your water intake throughout the day. Fruit juices, made to order in a blender with no additives, are good to have too. However, because of their sugar content, fruit juices should be your second choice. Minimize or avoid using fruits with a high-glycemic index, like grapes, apples or oranges because they contain too much sugar.

Natural stimulants like coffee are allowed, and you can add a trace of milk, preferably milk-foam. Most teas are okay, too. Make sure that the coffee and tea are not made with sugar or sugar substitutes, and don't add any. You don't want to trigger an insulin response or force your body to work harder as it attempts to detoxify chemical sweeteners. Every time you overtrigger the insulin response during the day, you block the process and can jeopardize the whole plan. Stay clear of all soft drinks.

I personally like to drink carrot and ginger juice. Sometimes I add beets or parsley to the mixture. It's delicious, detoxifying, and a very good source of active minerals and food enzymes which, as I've said before, are a top priority. The naturally occurring sugars in veggies (like carrots) are not simple, processed carbs, and the body can handle them very well.

You can have veggie juices every couple of hours. Drink them slowly, but within ten minutes after they are prepared to ensure that you'll receive all their live nutrients.

What to Eat

Fruits

In addition to freshly squeezed or blended fruit juices, eating whole fruits is also allowed and recommended (in moderation) during the Undereating Phase. Since you don't want to spike insulin, it is best to consume light, low-glycemic fruits that provide a lot of nutrition, such as berries (blueberries, blackberries, raspberries, strawberries, etc.). I highly recommend nutrition to sugar—meaning they contain a lot of minerals, vitamins, and flavones, but not much sugar. Some berries have healing properties and contain potent antioxidant properties, which are excellent for detoxifying, and they are believed to protect against cancer. They also complement the digestion of high-protein meals. Warriors ate berries seasonally during the day.

Eating an "apple a day" is another good choice during detoxification, as are pears. Tropical fruits, like papayas, mangoes, pineapples, as well as grapefruits, oranges, and kiwis are good, too. They are very dense fruits and contain lots of vitamins and enzymes.

"Live" (Raw) Vegetables

During the Undereating Phase you can eat raw, green vegetables, of any variety. They will detoxify without taxing too much insulin. Save the cooked vegetables for the Overeating Phase. If you really want to have cooked vegetables once in a while, it's best to have them steamed. Don't eat many because they can overload your system.

Live Enzymes—Rule of Nature

There's a rule in nature that all living foods contain their own self-digesting enzymes. When you process food, enzymes are destroyed, so the food moves through your system without digestive help, and it robs the natural enzyme pool of your body.

When the body is depleted of enzymes, it starts to compromise digestion. And when digestion is compromised, your health is compromised. That's the bottom line.

Live Minerals

The best accessible minerals are those naturally derived from live foods. These minerals are more potent, naturally ionized, and better assimilated by your body. For example, carrot juice is a wonderful natural supplier of live potent minerals and electrolytes, which alkalize and nourish your system instantly.

Natural minerals should taste good when you put them in your mouth. Wild animals lick salty rocks to ingest the minerals as they need them. In the past, people did, too. You'll be able to know whether you need minerals or not by your taste buds. As long as you're depleted of minerals, they'll taste good. Once enough is ingested, they no longer will. Synthetic minerals are another story. They taste like chemicals; therefore, you can't taste and balance them orally.

Having the right amount and balance of minerals in your system prevents food cravings. A deficiency of even one mineral may create a craving for a certain food. For instance, a zinc deficiency may create a craving (or even a deep, excruciating hunger) for protein, like meat and dairy, which are naturally high in zinc. Some people crave something—but they don't know what. It may well be due to a mineral deficiency.

Protein

If you feel it's necessary, you can eat a little protein. Remember, though, that you're detoxifying your body, so it's important to let your system rest—this is why I recommend minimizing protein intake during the Undereating Phase. To minimize the stress on your digestive system, use good quality lean protein that is easily digested, such as: sashimi, eggs, chicken breast, turkey breast, fish, shellfish, plain yogurt or kefir (low-fat or nonfat), cottage cheese, or whey protein. Don't mix proteins; and limit the amount to no more than 6 oz. You can also choose to have a handful of raw nuts, preferably almonds, instead of lean protein.

I like to use my own protein powder, Warrior Growth Serum, made from a proprietary blend of air-dried organic colostrum that has been taken from the first milk of a lactating cow, with other nutrients. Colostrum is the first fluid secreted by the mammary of a lactating mammal, just after a birth. Colostrum is believed to mimic the nutritional composition of human mother's milk and thus contains some unique immune supportive properties and growth factors which regular milk doesn't.

Protein Utilization

It's important for everyone who eats protein to understand protein utilization—especially so for athletes and bodybuilders who ingest so much protein to build their muscles.

The Undereating Phase of the Warrior Diet should potentiate your body to handle the Overeating Phase. One of the top priorities of the Warrior evening meal is protein, and proper protein assimilation is vital for your health.

Many athletes and bodybuilders reach a plateau, even though they exercise intensely and consume large amounts of protein daily. In my opinion, malabsorption of protein is the reason for this. With all the ads and information blitzed by the media, there's still much confusion regarding protein utilization. Without proper protein utilization, you cannot reach the peak anabolic state you need to build muscle and repair tissues. There's more to this, so bear with me.

Let's now cover these two essential issues regarding protein:

- Protein utilization
- The quality of protein consumed

Principles of Protein Utilization

The principal rules for protein utilization appear as a triangle. The top point is protein. On the lower left point of the triangle are enzymes and probiotics (the friendly bacteria in your intestinal tract), and on the right side is the live food factor. In this case I am referring to undenatured protein (protein which has not been denatured, broken or twisted). Protein should be minimally processed and not denatured.

This triangle is an organic structure, and each of the angles needs the other to be complete. Protein can never be fully digested without the help of enzymes, and enzymes cannot be completely potentiated without probiotics. To fully utilize protein you must optimize all three factors: enzymes, probiotics, and the live-food factor.

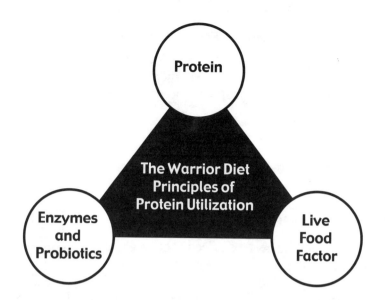

Protein Digestion (How It Works)

This is how it works. Protein, as you now know, needs digestive enzymes to be broken down. So, loading your body with enzymes is critical for protein utilization and digestion, especially if you ingest large amounts of protein. And, since a main function of probiotics is to break down the final waste and toxins into harmless substances, probiotics also help complete digestion and allow protein to be utilized more efficiently.

Carbohydrates

No carbohydrates, other than fresh vegetables and fruits, are allowed during the Undereating Phase. This includes bread, cereals, muffins, pastas, corn, potatoes, rice, barley, any other starchy foods, as well as candy, pastries, and all other sweets. None of these are allowed during the Undereating Phase*.

Go to "The Warrior Diet Daily Food Cycle" and "Lessons from History" (The Historical Role of Nutritional Carbohydrates) for information tailored to your specific needs.

Enzymes

Enzyme-Loading for Anti-aging

Research shows there's a connection between your body's pool of enzymes and your health. When your enzyme pool is loaded, enzymes run directly to your blood from the digestive tract and create a chain reaction of beneficial health effects, including antioxidant effects. Research has revealed that there is a link between your enzyme pool and aging. In other words, the fewer enzymes you have in your body the faster you age.

So, by reloading your body with enzymes, you may slow the aging cycle, rejuvenate your skin, and even reduce wrinkles. Enzyme reloading means ingesting more potent digestive enzymes than are actually needed for digestion, preferably on an empty stomach. Digestive enzymes act also as an intermediary in hormonal functions in your body. Reloading your body with live food enzymes will give you more vitality and will accelerate healing.

Burn Fat by Loading Your Body with Lipase

Research has shown that there's a link between a lipase deficiency (enzymes which break down fat) and obesity. Loading your body with lipase derived from live food—like raw avocados, raw nuts, and raw seeds—is one way to ensure proper fat metabolism and accelerate fat loss. Don't listen to those who tell you to avoid avocados or nuts because of their high-calorie, high-fat content. Quite the opposite. These foods in their raw state will help you to accelerate fat burning.

Note: It is best to consume high-fat raw foods, such as avocados and nuts, at night during the main meal so as not to overtax your system during the Undereating Phase. You may choose, however, to load your body with lipase during the Undereating Phase through enzyme supplementation.

SUPPLEMENTS FOR THE UNDEREATING PHASE

During the Undereating Phase you shouldn't overload your body with synthetic vitamins and minerals. If you choose to take supplements, make sure they're from a good source and made by a reliable company. Do your own research to make informed choices because taking the wrong supplements can hurt you. Some can be toxic just because they're not assimilated, and may be deposited in the wrong places. For example, taking excessive cheap supplemental calcium carbonate may cause calcium deposits in certain tissues and organs such as your joints and kidneys. Ideally, you can live quite well with proper nutrition and a minimum of supplements.

Nevertheless, there are some supplements that I often recommend people take during the "Undereating Phase:"

Digestive Enzymes

I believe strongly in the importance of digestive enzyme supplementation. Young people usually don't need them as much, but the older we get, the more necessary they often become. They're also helpful for athletes who eat more (usually protein) than the average person.

Digestive enzymes are vital to your health on a variety of levels:

1. Antioxidants

Research shows that in addition to breaking down food, digestive enzymes penetrate the blood and work almost like an antioxidant, destroying free radicals.

2. Anti-inflammatory

Protease enzymes (enzymes that break down protein) have anti-inflammatory properties, so people suffering from arthritis can benefit from them, as can those who experience inflammation in muscle tissue after a workout, or due to an injury. Enzymes (like bromelein) can prevent inflammation and injury, and reduce water retention.

3. Anti-allergenic

Many people suffer from food allergies and allergic reactions due to undigested food in the colon and blood. Undigested food creates inflammation, water retention, toxins, and slows down your whole system. Your body recognizes it as a foreign invader; thus triggering an allergic reaction. Digestive enzymes may help combat these problems.

4. Anti-cancerous

It's believed that overloading with digestive enzymes, especially when taken on an empty stomach, may assist in killing tumors and help prevent cancer.

Protease enzymes have unique properties, which go far beyond their digestive functions. You can find more about the therapeutic properties of digestive enzymes in the "Q&A" chapter.

5. Fat Burning

Loading your body with lipase may help accelerate fat metabolism and keep you lean.

Probiotics

Probiotics are the friendly (beneficial) bacteria in your digestive tract. They're necessary for healthy digestion and may be the first line of defense in disease prevention.

The main function of probiotics is to aid in the efficient absorption of food, vitamins, and minerals. They secrete antibiotic substances that destroy pathogenic (harmful) bacteria, yeast, and parasites, and thereby help you digest and assimilate your food (and thus use protein optimally).

The human gastrointestinal (GI) tract is supposed to contain 85 percent "good" bacteria and 15 percent "bad" bacteria. Unfortunately, many Westerners today have the opposite ratio. When our ancestors consumed fresh plant life hundreds and thousands of years ago they unknowingly ingested large amounts of these beneficial microorganisms. However, with the advent of modern farming techniques, which use chemicals such as pesticides, herbicides, and fungicides, these essential microorganisms have been greatly depleted from our food supply. Therefore, supplementation is often needed. For more information about probiotics, go to Warrior Probiotics in the "Warrior Nutritional Supplements" chapter.

Minerals

The most important supplements are minerals, especially if you exercise during the day, or are under stress. During the controlled-fasting time, especially when burning fat, toxins are released into the blood. Essential minerals will chelate (transport) a lot of the toxins out of your body and keep your hormonal levels intact. Live, potent minerals are also the first defense against radiation.

Unfortunately, mineral supplements don't seem to be a priority for most people, and the ignorance of them is stunning. Research indicates that many athletes and bodybuilders are deficient in several essential minerals like magnesium, potassium, calcium, and zinc.

Sometimes a deficiency occurs due to a mineral imbalance in the body. For example, if you take too much calcium, you may actually deplete your body of magnesium and zinc, and vice versa. Each mineral is essential for different bodily functions, and a deficiency in even one of them might lead to unpleasant symptoms and metabolic problems.

Magnesium deficiency is one of the main causes for tension headaches and nervousness. Zinc deficiency can cause chronic food cravings; copper deficiency might rob you of your sex drive. Chromium deficiency could cause insulin insensitivity that might lead to hyperglycemia, and possibly even diabetes in a later stage.

The list of mineral deficiencies is a long one. Most importantly, active people can deplete themselves of minerals in a matter of hours, especially during the summer months. When you practice controlled fasting, it's important to "max up" your minerals. Warriors in the past were aware of the essential role of minerals. Salt, for example, was a precious commodity and people used to trade mineral salts for gold.

I usually recommend taking a multimineral supplement that contains the right balance of minerals. Magnesium is essential not just for relaxing muscles and therefore avoiding muscle cramps and spasms, it's also necessary for maintaining hormonal levels, especially testosterone. Zinc is important for your glandular, reproductive, and immune systems. Active people especially need it. It's best to take the multimineral supplement before or right after your workout. Minerals alkalize your system and thus protect your body from the acidic side effects of physical and mental stress.

Note: Minerals should not make you nauseated if you use ones that are naturally derived from a live plant source. One of the best sources of minerals is coral-derived highly ionized minerals. Ionized minerals are biologically more active and better assimilated. For more on this, go to the "Warrior Nutritional Supplements" chapter.

Vitamins/Antioxidants/Herbs/Brain Boosters

Antioxidants

For extra protection against free radicals and to accelerate detoxification, there are certain vitamins and antioxidants that should be taken in the morning or during the day:

• Ester C with bioflavonoids. It is best to take vitamin C in the morning. (500-1000 milligrams).

• Grape seed extract is an antioxidant that is believed to be more potent than vitamin C or E, and can aid in the detoxification process and eliminate free radicals. (100-300 milligrams).

Antioxidant Treat

Another option is to take bilberry, blueberry, or elderberry powder. Take it out of the capsule and mix it with ½ teaspoon of raw honey. You can then mix this paste with water or chew it as is first thing in the morning. The purple pigment in berries, like bilberries, blueberries, blackberries, or elderberries is a most effective antioxidant. This is a natural alternative to popping grapeseed or pignogenol capsules, is much cheaper, and you can enjoy it while benefiting from it at the same time.

Multivitamins

Many people suffer from vitamin deficiencies. Stress, excessive alcohol consumption, smoking, and intense physical exercise may deplete your body from its B vitamins, vitamin C, E, and A. Taking a good quality multivitamin a day is a way to ensure an adequate vitamin supply in your body. Nevertheless, I recommend that people take a few extras as well, simply because the dosage amounts of certain vitamins (such as vitamin C) in some multivitamins are too low. You can take the multivitamin in the morning or at night with your main meal. Those who workout in the morning, or during the day, may want to take a multivitamin afterwards, because exercise depletes essential vitamins from the body.

All of my suggestions for supplemental stimulants and herbs, are optional.

Ginseng (Panax and Siberian)

Ginseng is an adaptogenic herb, meaning an herb that helps you to adapt to stress. I find ginseng to be a good natural stimulator and substitute for those who are sensitive to caffeine. I like to alternate between these two natural stimulants (ginseng and caffeine) so that I don't overdo either of them.

Ginseng could be especially helpful during the Undereating Phase. Besides being a wonderful aid against stress, it also contains antioxidant and healing properties. Both ginseng and ginkgo biloba are believed to be aphrodisiac herbs. They boost the body's own production of nitric oxide (NO). Nitric oxide plays a vital role in regulating blood pressure. Moreover, nitric oxide is essential for getting and maintaining erections and for sexual potency. This ancient herb (ginseng) has been used for thousands of years. Today, scientists believe it contains more beneficial properties that still need to be researched.

I like to mix ginseng with ½ teaspoon of raw honey. I use panax during the day or Siberian ginseng at night. I enjoy the taste and aroma of this bittersweet herb. The honey makes it more edible and I believe it helps in the delivery of its nutrients. (Panax is a pick-up herb, while Siberian ginseng is more of a sedative).

Ginger

Ginger is a warming thermogenic herb with anti-inflammatory properties, and one of the best natural digestive aids. Gingerol, the active ingredient in ginger, possesses natural antibiotic properties, which makes it a wonderful herb for detoxification.

I mix ginger powder (200-500 milligrams) with a ½ teaspoon of rice syrup. It tastes like a hot candy, freshens your breath, cleans your mouth and warms your body. I have this during the day. I also like tto add fresh ginger to the veggie juices I drink during the Undereating Phase.

Brain Boosters

There are natural ways to boost brain neurotransmitters throughout the Undereating Phase. The "empty-stomach factor" can accelerate the delivery of certain amino acids and nutrients to the brain. By crossing the brain barrier, these nutrients can boost mood, alleviate depression, and give you a feeling of well-being.

Glutamine

Glutamine is a free-form amino acid that nourishes your brain as a daily fuel. The main fuel for the brain is glucose, but when glucose supply is short, the brain converts glutamine into glucose and uses it as a reserve fuel. Glutamine also works as a neurotransmitter boosting the feeling of well-being and assertiveness.

The Undereating Phase is the best time to take glutamine supplements. When you take this amino acid on an empty stomach, it will cross the brain barrier and do its job as a brain booster. However, when glutamine is taken with food, it won't reach the brain. The body will use it as fuel, or to replenish the lining of the digestive tract. Glutamine is believed to be a stress-hormone blocker. On top of all this, Glutamine is essential for the anabolic process. This protein is found in very high concentration in the muscle tissue. Every time you are under physical stress, your muscles lose glutamine. Chronic depletion of glutamine may lead to a catabolic process of losing muscle tissues. Maintaining a proper diet should be adequate to supply your body's demand for glutamine. Nevertheless, it's worth considering glutamine supplementation during the day if you want to boost your mind and muscle performance. As I've said before, use the advantage of the empty-stomach factor through the Undereating Phase to ensure maximum glutamine absorption.

Ginkgo Biloba, Tyrosine, and DMAE

I personally like to take ginkgo biloba to increase circulation, especially in the brain, and to enhance memory. Additionally,

Tyrosine and DMAE may boost your dopamine and acetylcholine (major brain neurotransmitters) if you take them on an empty stomach.

Boosting your dopamine will improve your mood, making you more alert and excited to face the day. High dopamine is linked to an increase of growth hormone. In an indirect way, dopamine keeps testosterone levels high by blocking prolactin (the hormone that stimulates milk production).

A complete list of recommended nutritional supplements can be found in the "Warrior Diet Nutritional Supplements" chapter.

PROTEIN POWDERS— A REVIEW

For athletes or bodybuilders who are interested in keeping their protein consumption high during the day, protein powders could be an instant alternative to cooked meals. However, it's very important to choose the right one. Protein powders are divided into three groups: dairy, soy, and egg.

Whey Protein

Whey (a dairy protein) is considered by many nutritionists to be one of the best powders for its immuno-supportive properties. It's also a complete protein food. Ideally, a good whey protein powder is supposed to contain two factors to make it alive and potent:

1. Immunoglobulins—proteins that support the immune system by containing IgA and IgE, which trigger immunity antigenic activity against pathogens and infections.

2. Growth factors—that translate in your body as growth hormone derivatives, good at promoting tissue repair, growth and rejuvenation.

Commercial Whey Protein

Unfortunately, most commercial whey protein manufacturers compromise on the immunoglobulins (the protein that supports the immune system). And, as far as I know, none contain any growth factors. Growth factors (especially IGF-1) are bound to the fat globules of the raw dairy. High-temperature processing, pasteurization, and removal of the fat completely eviscerates commercial whey powders of growth factors, as well as their pharmaceutical potency.

To top it all, many of these powders are loaded with estrogenic substances and chemicals. The beef and dairy industries use estrogenic hormones to increase cattle weight. Prolactin (a milk-producing hormone) is sometimes added to the drug mixture to stimulate milk production. Prolactin has a devastating blocking effect on testosterone. Derivatives of all these toxins may appear in the milk and products that are derived from milk, unless they're made from organic milk. Do your own research. Look for products from reliable manufacturers and suppliers, and check the processing methods and ingredients used.

Lactoferin, the Magic Bullet

Lactoferin is a major immune supportive protein in an infant's mother's milk that protects babies from bacterial infections. It's also the best iron scavenger. Lactoferin is abundant in good quality colostrums and whey protein, but it rarely appears in commercial dairy protein powders. This is too bad, because in addition to its iron scavenging abilities, lactoferin deposits iron in places where the body really needs it. Iron oxidation is a tremendous problem, not just because it can toxify the tissues, but also because it feeds the bad bacteria in your intestinal tract, such as bacteria that cause yeast infections.

Some researchers believe that lactoferin has anticancerous properties, and scientists surmise that lactoferin contains other healing properties, including that it may eventually combat chronic diseases such as AIDS and cancer. However, these issues need further research. Nevertheless, based on current data, lactoferin could be one of the most promising "dairy derivative" healing aids in the future.

Dairy Protein Powders

Regrettably, whey protein powders are not the only protein powders with problems. Most dairy protein powders on the market today are just not "clean." For instance, dairy protein powders (the most highly consumed protein powders) are generally produced cheaply with overaggressive processing methods. As a result, they often contain denatured protein and toxic byproducts.

This can have a terrible effect on your body. Besides being toxic, what's possibly most upsetting is that some of this denatured protein is deposited in body tissues, compromising the integrity of the tissue fibers, and may eventually damage lean tissues in your muscles or skin.

Pasteurization alone can cause negative potential side effects. The process separates the milk from the friendly bacteria within it, which is killed by the heat. The acidity of pasteurized dairy also increases to the point that it's no longer natural (raw milk has neutral to alkaline pH). Since raw (unpasteurized) milk is illegal in the United States, the only alternative I know of is low-temperature processed, freeze or air-dried pasteurized dairy powders, which retain most ingredients in their natural state.

Warrior Growth Serum

Since commercially available protein powders today are so denuded of growth factors and immuno-supportive factors, and most lack lactoferin, I decided a few years ago to work on producing a potent, natural dairy protein myself that does contain all these missing potent factors. After much research, trial and error, and with the help of some trusted friends, this powder, which I call "Warrior Growth Serum," was finally produced. It's designed to mimic human mother's milk. I believe "Warrior Growth Serum" is the most potent protein powder that exists today, and the best dairy powder that, as far as I know, has ever existed. Moreover, the taste is so superb that people who try chewing it (yes, chew the raw powder!) find themselves bingeing on it. Some people have told me that it reminds them of an old, delicious taste they haven't experienced for years.

I use "Warrior Growth Serum" powder during the Undereating/ fasting period — especially before and after my workout. More on this ultimate protein, as well as other protein powders that can help you accelerate your anabolic and metabolic states—all aimed at getting your body adapted to the Warrior Diet — can be found in the "Warrior Diet Nutritional Supplements."

Soy Protein Powders

I don't use soy protein powders. There are several reasons why:

• Pasteurized processed soy powder loses a lot of its nutritional value when compared to the whole soybeans.

• Soy protein is high in protein-inhibitor substances, like phytates, which may also inhibit mineral digestion. The Undereating Phase requires that you only eat protein that's easily assimilated. Processed soy may have negative effects on the thyroid gland. An under-active thyroid leads to slow metabolism, fatigue, and impotence.

• Soy protein contains some properties that may accelerate estrogenic effects for some people. Soy flavones are estrogen-like substances that may trigger estrogen-related symptoms in people who are sensitive to soy.

• Many people are sensitive to soy. Soy is one of the most allergenic foods, especially when it's highly processed.

• Most soy powder supplements are loaded with fillers and gums that may irritate your guts, and cause bloating and pain.

• The fiber in textured vegetable soy protein is harsh and tough on your system. I don't recommend it for anyone who has a sensitive digestive tract.

This said, sometimes I like to have whole soybeans (edamame) during the Overeating Phase as a complementary source of protein from whole food.

Egg-Protein Powders

I personally do not consume commercial egg-protein powders. However, whole organic eggs are a very good source of protein, minerals, vitamins, and essential fatty acids. Therefore, I recommend consuming eggs, mainly for the Overeating Phase, but once in a while it's okay to eat eggs during the Undereating Phase. Make sure that you consume the whole egg, with the yolk, and that they are organic eggs. Bodybuilders and athletes who like to consume egg whites only as a source of protein should try to keep a ratio of about four to six egg whites to one yolk. The yolk contains many vitamins and vital nutrients, so don't skip it.

Summary of the Undereating Phase

Once you have finished the Undereating Phase, you've kept to the priorities of detoxification. You did your enzyme-loading, optimized your glandular and hormonal systems, and stabilized your insulin. You turned your body—naturally—into a fat-burning machine.

It's best to exercise now to accelerate these effects even further. But, since the Warrior Diet is, after all, a diet, I'll complete the diet section first, and we will deal with exercise in the "Warrior Workout" chapter. Besides, you may only wish to incorporate the diet components into your life. I strongly believe that a very good way to start on the Warrior Diet is by following the diet elements first. This alone will probably do the job. Moreover, it may stimulate even sedentary people to begin some kind of physical activity, due to all the extra energy people generally feel when they become warriors.

In the next chapter you're going to learn how to practice the Overeating Phase of the Warrior Diet.

FOODS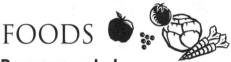

Recommended:

- Live (raw) fruits and vegetables
- Freshly prepared fruits and vegetable juices
- Warrior Growth Serum

Optional:

- Small amount of lean protein
- Handful of raw almonds

SUPPLEMENTS

Recommended:

- Vitamin C
- Grapeseed extract
- Coral-derived highly ionized minerals
- Probiotics
- Enzymes
- Multivitamin (may be taken at night)

Optional:

- Ginseng
- Gingko Biloba
- Ginger
- Glutamine
- Tyrosine
- DMAE

CHAPTER FIVE
THE OVEREATING
PHASE

Overeating generally means eating more than normal. But what is normal? When people refer to the term "normal" they usually think it relates to a standard that all should live by. However, what many people call "sensible eating" doesn't always make sense to me. And, in my mind "normal" isn't a clear-cut indication of quality. I feel it's high time to reconsider and reevaluate the concept of overeating. I'll explain why and how overeating can work for you in short order.

You've now reached the point that it's time to eat your main meal. Your body is conditionally depleted of carbohydrates. Your hormonal levels are at their height, and their effects are accelerated even more if you've just exercised. Your growth hormone has picked up, and your enzyme pool is fully loaded. Most important, your insulin level is at peak sensitivity, which is one of the biggest advantages of the Warrior Diet.

Put simply, your body is ready now to consume large amounts of food without gaining body fat. This is the best time to eat as much as you want and enjoy this wonderful sense of freedom.

The Overeating Principles

Overeating sounds like a lot of fun. As a matter of fact, it is! But there is an order to this "piggin' out" thing. In other words, you have to know *how to overeat* during your main meal.

The Overeating Principles are based on Three Rules of Eating:

Rule #1: Always start with subtle-tasting foods and move to the more aggressive.

Rule #2: Include as many tastes, textures, colors, and aromas as possible in your main meal.

Rule #3: Stop eating when you feel much more thirsty than hungry.

I highly recommend that you start with veggies, and then move to protein and carbs. To fully enjoy your meal, try to prepare the food in a way that will incorporate as many tastes, textures, colors, and aromas as possible. Finally, you should be able to stop eating instinctively—either when you feel pleasantly satisfied, or when you become significantly more thirsty than hungry.

There is of course much more to it, but once you understand these basic rules, you can practice the Overeating Phase and reach the goals of this phase of the diet. Part two of this chapter goes into more detail on these three rules.

Instinctual Eating

The Overeating Phase does not involve guilt or obsessive self-control. You should find that by following the rules you'll create a way of eating that is more instinctive. By trusting your instincts, you'll experience a sense of freedom and real satisfaction. Having a sense of freedom, as I've said before, is necessary to be truly happy.

The Goals of Overeating

- Accelerate your anabolism (repairing tissues and building muscles)
- Boost your metabolism
- Replenish your glycogen reserves
- Nourish your body and mind for pleasure and full satisfaction (compensation)
- While eating, experience a sense of freedom (guilt-free)
- Retrain to eat instinctively

Part One
Controlled Overeating

The Science Behind Overeating

I'd like to address the issue of overeating. This is a controversial idea. It should make sense once you read it, so please keep reading.

Briefly, what happens when people practice overeating after controlled fasting is that their body changes to a more thermogenic and highly metabolized state. In other words, your brain receives a signal that it should elevate metabolism in order to burn these extra calories. On the whole, when one overeats after a controlled fast, nutrients are assimilated at a greater rate, there is an acceleration of the anabolic process of repairing tissues and building muscles, depleted glycogen reserves are replenished, there's an increased secretion of adrenal hormones, thyroid hormones, and an elevation of androgenic hormones (sex hormones, such as testosterone). If overeating is practiced regularly, your body's metabolism will remember this, and with adaptation to these daily high-calorie meals, should become metabolically faster and more efficient than before.

Here's the good news: it's fairly simple to retrain your taste buds. As noted, after the Undereating Phase, your taste buds are very fresh, so that's the best time to train yourself to acquire subtle tastes.

Exploring the Advantages of Overeating

1. Metabolic Acceleration Per Meal

Scientific studies say that there's a correlation between our metabolism and how many calories are consumed per day. However, as far as I know, no studies have been conducted on the correlation between our metabolism and the amount of calories consumed per meal. I truly believe that the amount of calories consumed per meal is the bottom line.

2. Adaptation to High-Calorie Meals (Metabolic Acceleration)

Let me give you an example of how adaptation works. Take, for instance, a workout. People can walk for two hours and not build muscle, but can sprint for only five minutes and build muscles and endurance. So, it's not necessarily the length of time spent exercising, it's the intensity of the exercise. Coming back to the subject of diet, the question remains: Is it the intensity of the meal that will dictate your body's metabolism? My answer is yes. That's the way I experience it.

3. Overeating: A Primal Instinct

The Warrior Diet is the only diet that explores the advantages of overeating. I want to say something to all those who overeat and then feel guilty. You feel guilty because you didn't know that a deep, primal instinct drove you to overeat. Many people binge late at night when exhausted from a rigid, obsessive, daily self-control. That's usually the time when inhibitions are broken down and the alleged "demons" come out. But these are not demons. If you know how to use this instinct in the right way, it can work for you instead of against you.

Part Two
The Three Rules of Eating

First Rule: *Always Start with Subtle-Tasting Foods and Move to More Aggressive-Tasting Foods*

Start with raw veggies, then move to protein and cooked veggies, and finish with carbohydrates.

It's okay to combine protein and carbohydrates. However, if your goal is to lose weight, have the carbohydrates at the end of your meal. Following this method can also prove effective for those who like to rotate between high protein days and high carbohydrate days.

Subtle Tastes

The first rule of eating is to start with subtle tastes (the tastes that nature gave us—free of processed, fried foods, and sugar). If you start with foods that have more aggressive tastes and then move back to more subtle ones, your body won't react as well.

Everyone can develop a subtle taste, and it's very important to do so. After a controlled fast, you already start to develop a subtle taste, and the foods that possess the subtlest tastes are actually raw vegetables. Soon after starting the Warrior Diet, you should find that you'll begin to enjoy eating raw (living) vegetables.

The American diet is too aggressive—too much sugar, salt, fried fats, and overly processed foods. It's hard to enjoy natural food when one is used to aggressive tastes. In the past, food was more natural and subtle. People didn't have access to refined sugar. Honey was scarce. I believe the human body is basically built for subtle, whole-food tastes. But taste buds today have been dulled from being fed an aggressive, overly processed diet from an early age.

If you choose to consume more natural food, you'll develop a subtle taste rather quickly and will begin to find it unappealing to eat foods that are too aggressive. Even after just a few months people tell me that they no longer crave fast-food meals. This is the truth; they say that they'd rather have salad greens, steamed veggies, a stew, broiled fish, chicken, or a steak.

How to Begin the Overeating Phase and Follow the First Rule

Begin the Overeating Phase with live (raw), leafy green vegetables. The greener they are, the better they are, and the denser they are the better it is. Starting with a mixed green salad is a good choice. A handful of parsley, a cucumber, and some endive leaves can be added to your salad as well as other vegetables, like tomatoes, raw onion, scallions, and olives. They'll enhance flavor, texture, and the salad's nutritional composition. The amount to consume is optional. Use your instincts.

There are several reasons to start the meal with live food (raw vegetables):

- Your stomach lining is very sensitive, and when you first ingest dead food, it doesn't react so well.

- Vitamins and minerals are absorbed more quickly when live (raw) greens are the first thing to reach the stomach.

- It's also healthy for the digestive system since raw foods are high in food enzymes, which are vital for optimum digestion and elimination.

If you prefer to have a low-glycemic fruit, such as berries, grapefruit, or a tropical fruit such as a papaya, mango, or pineapple as an appetizer, this is also allowed. Tropical fruits are good because they're very dense and contain a lot of digestive enzymes. As a general rule though, I'd rather you begin the Overeating Phase with leafy greens.

Second Rule: *Include As Many Tastes, Textures, Colors, and Aromas As Possible in Your Main Meal*

It's my strong belief that you should try to include as many different tastes, textures, colors, and aromas as possible in your main meal because doing so will deliver a complete feeling of satiety. If you miss even one of them on a regular basis, after a while you'll probably develop food cravings.

Aside from hot and cold, warm and cool, sweet and sour, salty and bitter, spicy and plain, tart, pungent, and astringent (the sharp, biting or harsh taste in foods, such as that in ginger and hot radishes), we know there are other factors, like aromas, colors, and textures, which also relate to and affect taste, and are vital to feeling satiety.

- *Tastes:* sweet, sour, salty, bitter, spicy, astringent, pungent, smoked
- *Textures:* hard, soft, crunchy, sticky, grainy, chunky, smooth, chewy, jelly, gummy, light, heavy, thick, thin, wet, and dry
- *Aromas:* are related to all of the above, such as sweet, sharp, smoked, rich, aged—like cheeses or wine
- *Colors*: green, orange, red, yellow, purple, brown, white, black, blue
- *Temperatures:* hot, warm, room-temperature, cool, cold, frozen

---

The more variety you introduce in your diet the better off you'll be. There are enormous possibilities. When preparing meals, you should try to incorporate this huge variety as much as possible. Combining them in the right balance is the art of cooking. Traditionally, meals were prepared like this. (See "Lessons From History," chapter 7, for more on this.)

Sensing Essential Nutrients

Different foods contain different essential nutrients. Your body can instinctively sense essential nutrients by sight, smell, taste, and touch (textures), and they activate pleasure sensors in your brain. There is a connection between cravings and nutrient deficiencies. For example, people who suffer from a mineral deficiency often crave salty foods, and those on a very low carbohydrate diet often develop cravings for sweet foods.

Some natural foods, such as mother's milk, contain all the tastes necessary to satisfy a newborn baby. Natural foods that contain all the tastes are usually the most nourishing. The main idea here is to prepare a meal that contains as many tastes, aromas, colors, and textures as possible, so one can reach full satisfaction and at the same time nourish oneself with all the essential nutrients.

Colors and Nutrition

The pigmentation in foods marks the presence of vital nutrients, flavones, minerals, or vitamins. There are different theories about how to combine food colors. Some suggest to start the day with bright colors, such as yellow, orange, and red, and to finish the day with purple, black, and brown. Others believe that there's a correlation between the color of food and different inner energies. According to this theory, red stimulates sexual energy, while yellow and orange are spiritual energizers. Regardless, colors should never be taken for granted. This is one way of evaluating the nutritional quality of whole foods. Introducing a variety of colors in a meal will enhance the nutritional composition. It's also aesthetically pleasing and helps you reach satiety.

Third Rule: *Stop Eating When You Feel Much More Thirsty Than Hungry*

How Do You Know When You Reach Satiety?

A lot of people say, "I eat and eat and never reach satiety." Well, on the Warrior Diet you're going to reach satisfaction. And the more you practice it, the more you will feel satisfied.

First of all, you're allowed to eat as much as you want, so you don't eat feeling guilty. And, the minute you start to become more thirsty than hungry, that's the first indication that satisfaction is coming. It means that you now need more water than food, and it's time to start thinking about finishing. Allowing your thirst to become a parameter for controlling your satiety is an instinctual matter. When you drink after dinner, you probably won't want to eat after that, because you'll feel like you gave your body exactly what it desired, and any more is unnecessary.

But if you're still hungry, you can eat again. There is no rule to stop. You're not going to gain body fat because, as I said, your insulin is at peak sensitivity, and your body is busy replenishing your depleted glycogen reserves.

You might get tired after eating your meal. Use this time for relaxation——read, watch TV, wash dishes, or do nothing, just as long as it makes you feel peaceful. However, it's best to wait at least two hours after finishing the meal before going to bed.

A Few Words on Hunger and Thirst

Your body has more sensitivity, in general, to hunger than to thirst. There is a common presumption that there's a sort of defect in our sense of thirst, so we often don't drink as much as we need to. In my opinion, one of the reasons why some people lack thirst-sensitivity is because if we were thirsty all the time, we simply wouldn't eat as much as we need to. And for active people this could be fatal.

Regardless, people who lack the ability to sense thirst are in constant danger of dehydration. Dehydration, as most know, can lead to headaches, fever, kidney stones, high-blood pressure, and even death.

It is believed that when you force yourself to drink on a daily basis, it helps develop a greater sense of actual thirst. Soldiers in the army go through this. When I was in the army, I remember being told to stand in line and drink a couple of liters of water before training.

Let me note here that those who fail to supply their bodies with enough water put themselves in danger of compromising all metabolic systems. Without enough water, nutrient assimilation plummets, toxins are not eliminated, and the fat-burning process slows down. It's commonly recommended that adults drink at least 6–8 glasses of water per day; however, in my opinion you should try to gradually increase your intake beyond this amount, especially throughout the day, and during and after a workout. (I personally drink between one to two liters of water during and after my workout). Starting your day with a glass or two of pure water (with lemon, if you like it) is a great way to begin the detoxification and elimination process.

How to Instinctively Stop Eating

For those who have large appetites and don't instinctively know when to stop eating, here's my answer: once you reach the point that you feel significantly more thirsty than hungry. That's when to start drinking. I'm probably the first one to tell you that the time to stop eating is not when you count your calories and say, "If I eat more I'm going to gain weight." And it's not because somebody told you to count the macro and micro nutrition. Stay away from all this guilt. You can eat unlimited amounts from all the groups discussed. But when your body tells you it's more thirsty than hungry (and it will tell you more and more as you practice the Warrior Diet), this is the time to stop.

Take a break and drink a glass of water or cup of tea. If after 15 or 20 minutes you still feel hungry, you can eat again. You probably won't be, but if you still are, go ahead and eat again. No other diet will give you this freedom.

What to Drink After the Main Meal

In addition to water, any tea that stimulates digestion is good. Herb teas, such as peppermint, ginger, green and chamomile are highly recommended. I often like to drink ginger tea or green tea mixed with ginger tea. The nights when my main meal is largely protein, I like to sweeten my tea with a natural sweetener like raw honey or maple syrup. Sweetened teas may help stop sugar cravings and enhance your feeling of satiety.

Other beverages, such as regular or decaf coffee, cappuccino, latte, espresso, or even hot chocolate, are also okay to have. Treat them like a dessert.

Coming up in the next chapter, you'll learn "everything you wanted to know but were afraid to ask" about the main evening meal.

Chapter Six
THE MAIN MEAL:
Food Preparations
for the Overeating
Phase

This chapter is all about the main meal. It covers every aspect—from choosing foods and food preparations to food reviews. Also included: what's good, what's bad, and what's ugly (meaning not so bad, but not so good either.)

The Importance of Choosing Fresh Foods

Choosing fresh foods is part of the "Warrior Instinct." Predators are very conscientious about the food they eat. A wild cat first smells, licks, and then eats its food. If the food doesn't smell or taste right, the cat won't touch it. The survival of these animals depends upon their ability to distinguish between fresh and stale foods, and the same could be said about warriors.

Cooking Your Own Meals (to follow the second rule of eating)

I'm a big believer in cooking your own meals. I feel that cooking celebrates self-respect, and it's especially important on the Warrior Diet. Through cooking, you can control exactly what you put inside your body. It's a creative process, where you use trial and error to determine exactly what you like, and can use different herbs and spices to increase or balance flavors, aromas, and textures. You're not a scavenger on the Warrior Diet. You work to purchase (gather) the food, prepare, and cook it. Controlling the entire process is very important. For more on Warrior recipes, see the "Warrior Meals and Recipes" chapter.

Advantages of Eating Cooked, Warm Food

People have consumed warm food since the discovery of fire. Yet there's a lack of awareness today about the important role that temperature plays in the food that we eat.

The main meal of the Warrior Diet encourages consumption of cooked, warm food, especially since the Undereating Phase is based mostly on raw (live) uncooked foods. I know there are people who preach that we should only eat raw food, but with all due respect, I disagree with them.

There are several advantages to consuming cooked, warm food:

- Eating warm food often brings more satisfaction than cold food. The thermogenic (warming) effect slightly increases the temperature in your brain so you feel more satisfied and happy with your meal.
- Warm temperatures are beneficial for your digestive tract. The digestive tract reacts much more efficiently to warm than to cold food. Food is easier to digest when warm.
- Some people are sensitive to cold foods; others suffer from overacidity. Well-cooked warm food may help deal with these issues.
- Warm food stimulates the immune system.
- More of the flavones bound to the fiber of many veggies and certain fruits are released, and can be better absorbed, when they're cooked.

Warm Food—Like a Fresh Kill

I strongly believe that eating warm food mimics the effect of a fresh kill. A predator's first bite of its prey always tastes warm (since this is a fresh kill). Scavengers, on the other hand, who eat leftover corpses, enjoy the cold taste of the animal that was killed by a predator beforehand. It's my belief that when you eat and enjoy warm food, it triggers the Predator Instinct, and those people who settle with cold leftovers may trigger the Scavenger Instinct.

Napoleon and the Predator Instinct

Eating chicken with your hands can indicate a Predator Instinct. Napoleon was notorious during his war campaigns for tearing apart a whole, cooked chicken and eating it with his hands. It's interesting to note that the night before Waterloo, Napoleon changed this habit and ate fried potatoes. As you probably know, Napoleon lost that battle.

Go and Kill a Pizza

Please indulge me for a moment and let's look at hot pizza in a completely different way. The crust is dry and, to me, it resembles the skin of a hunted animal; the inside is soft and warm, with melted cheese and red tomato sauce that's like the warm blood and flesh of a fresh kill; the way pizza is eaten mimics the way people used to hold fresh meat in their hands and, yes, bite the bloody thing. To continue with this line of thinking, I could even argue that eating fresh pizza is like a virtual reality of a bloody kill. This may sound appalling to you. Or it may not. In either case, next time you're in the mood, go and hunt for a fresh pizza. The Warrior Diet doesn't recommend eating pizza often, but once in a while it's okay to have a slice or two.

Cooking Vegetables to Optimize Flavors and Flavones

Cooked vegetables possess different tastes, textures, and aromas. Certain veggies like parsley, celery, and cilantro work like herbs and spices to enhance the flavors and nutritional composition of a meal.

Vegetables are like water; you can have as much of them as you want. These calories don't count.

Now let's be specific. Other than leafy greens and salad foods, for the main course, the veggies should be cooked. Besides the advantages listed above, cooking, as noted, also frees more of the flavones from the veggies.

1. Tomatoes

Only a small percentage of the lycopene (an important carotene flavone) in tomatoes is absorbed when eating raw tomatoes. That doesn't mean it's bad to eat fresh tomatoes, but when you cook them you greatly increase lycopene absorption.

2. Broccoli and Cauliflower

Indole-3 carbinol, found in broccoli, cauliflower, and all cruciferous vegetables, is a very important flavone, which is bound to the protein of the fiber. When you eat cruciferous vegetables in their raw state, this flavone can hardly be absorbed. These vegetables need to be cooked in order to potentiate flavone assimilation, whether they're inside the veggie or on the fiber. Moreover, vegetables such as broccoli and cauliflower taste better when cooked.

Indole-3 carbinol helps both men and women protect against estrogenic effects. Indole-3 carbinol is believed to help the liver detoxify estrogen derivatives, protect against cancer, and may cosmetically make you look leaner.

3. Berries

Cooking berries potentiates their flavones to a much higher degree. However, it may destroy live enzymes as well as some vitamins. The natural balance of nutrients is changed when you cook the raw fruit.

4. Legumes and Grains

Another substance that has been the subject of much current research is IP6, inositol hexaphosphate. Researchers believe today that IP6, found in the fiber of legumes and grains, is the major ingredient responsible for preventing colon cancer and other cancers. Food must be well cooked in order to free IP6 from the fiber and enable it to be absorbed in the system.

IP6 seldom appears in soluble fiber. It's usually attached to the bran, the hard (insoluble) fiber, which is difficult to digest. IP6 is found in legumes, peas, wheat, barley, and oats.

Raw versus Cooked Veggies in the Main Meal

Ideally, leafy green veggies should be eaten raw. They should cause no problem with digestion even if you consume a fair amount of them. But, as just stated, cruciferous vegetables, like broccoli, cauliflower, kale, and Brussels sprouts, should be cooked. There's no reason to eat them raw. You won't be able to assimilate as many nutrients if you eat them raw and they're not going to taste as good either. Moreover, when eating them raw, you'll likely suffer from unpleasant symptoms like gas and bloating.

Some raw plants may cause toxicity. Most sprouts, for instance, need to be soaked and washed well to remove toxins or other substances that may block nutrient absorption. Alfalfa sprouts should be eaten only when the sprouts reach maturity of at least three days. They should look green. If eaten prematurely, alfalfa sprouts may be toxic.

High-Sulfur Foods

Some foods are high in the mineral sulfur. As mentioned before, high-sulfur proteins like cysteine work as antioxidants, and can be helpful as a defense against cancer and radiation. Cysteine is necessary for optimum metabolism, and is destroyed by aggressive processing and heat.

Sulfur is a mineral and a gas-forming substance. Be aware of how you combine high-sulfur foods when cooking. For examples, eggs are high-sulfur protein. When you eat eggs and cabbage, or eggs and cauliflower, or eggs and broccoli, you might suffer from bloating and gas because these veggies are high-sulfur foods, too, and you may be consuming too much at once. So be careful about combinations and quantities, and try to incorporate different types of foods, not only one group at a time. If you really want to combine high-sulfur foods, let your body adjust slowly to this.

If you suffer from sulfite sensitivity, you should consider supplementing with molybendum, a trace mineral, which is involved in sulfite metabolism.

Foods Containing High-Sulfur Proteins:

Eggs

Raw milk

Raw Cheese

Colostrum

Low-temperature, processed whey

High-Sulfur Vegetables:

Broccoli

Cabbage

Cauliflower

Kale

Brussels Sprouts

Spinach

Eggplant

Cooked eggplant goes very well with protein meals, such as meat and fish. The soft, oily texture of peeled, cooked eggplant balances the harder, meaty texture of the protein (especially after you trim the fat off the meat). When mixed together it gives the meat natural tenderness and adds more texture to the meal.

Squash

I highly recommend eating all of the squash family. They contain numerous nutrients and minerals, and are wonderful for the digestive tract. I actually think the squash family is among the very best for the digestive tract. Squash aid in the elimination process without gas or bloating. They should be cooked well. There's no reason to eat squash raw.

Soups and Stews

I'm a big believer in soups and stews, not just in cold seasons, but even in warm weather. I think having veggies and soup is one of the best ways to start a meal. Hearty vegetable soups and stews, where everything is cooked together—often veggies, roots, meats or seafood, and whole grains—have a great advantage in that many tastes, textures, and aromas combine in one hearty, hot meal. This thousand's-of-years-old tradition is extremely good for your satiety. Fermented soups (like miso soup) are also great. Miso is a natural alkalizer. Fermented foods are helpful for your digestion and the balance of healthy bacteria in your guts.

Protein

Proteins bear different tastes, textures, colors, and aromas. Dominant textures are chewy, wet, dry, hard, soft, or creamy. Dominant tastes are sweet, salty, and pungent.

After veggies, what the body needs most (second among the subtle tastes) is protein. When you're hungry, starving, or lost in the jungle, the first thing that your body needs is protein. Human beings can survive without carbohydrates, yet cannot survive without complete protein. Complete protein foods contain all the essential amino acids. The body can synthesize carbohydrates from protein or fat; however, the body can't produce essential amino acids without ingesting it from outside sources. Therefore, in order to survive, the body needs complete protein. Both women and men should make protein their top priority.

Meat, Poultry, and Fish

While being on the Warrior Diet, you're going to crave for exactly the things you need most. After going through the Undereating Phase, people crave protein. It doesn't have to be meat or fish. It may be beans, nuts, legumes, or cheese. For active men particularly, I feel there's no substitute for whole protein that comes from organic fresh meat, especially if you trim away the fat and cook it properly. Animal proteins should always be lean.

The exception to this is fish. In principle, fish oils (fat) are very healthy. I do have some concern about them, however, because a lot of fish today is contaminated due to polluted waters, and most of the toxins are in their fat tissues. Please don't misunderstand me here. Fish is an excellent source of protein. It's high in organic iodine, and is an excellent natural source of essential fatty acids (EFA's) in their most active form, EPA and DHA. These EFA derivatives are essential for brain development and maintenance, and are the building blocks for prostaglandins and the hormonal system.

The least-contaminated fish, I believe, are low-fat white fish such as flounder, sole, or turbot.

> Research continues to show that men who are meat eaters have much more virility, while those who are purely vegetarian have reduced testosterone levels, potency, and sperm count. Part of the reason for this is that many vegetarians simply don't know how to practice food combining and suffer from protein deficiency as well as a deficiency of certain vitamins, such as B12, and vital minerals such as zinc, calcium, and iron.

Organic Proteins— "Say No To Drugs"

I recommend buying organic proteins to avoid the hazardous effects of hormones, antibiotics, pesticides, and other toxins such as rendered feed (ground-up remains of dead animals, including "road kill") that some meat growers use. Organic proteins also taste better. They're accessible today and, granted, cost a little more; but it's worth it.

Farm-raised fish can be healthier, but recent research has shown that they may also contain contaminants. So right now it's pretty much a toss up whether farm-raised or free-swimming fish is better for you.

Eggs

Eggs have different tastes and textures. The dominant tastes are sweet and salty, and textures soft, smooth, wet, or oily.

Eggs are another good source of protein. Don't be afraid to eat the egg yolk. It's a natural supplement of vitamins A to E, and the essential sulfur-containing protein cysteine. The yellow pigment of the yolk is a vital carotene, so don't eat just the egg whites. For those who consume many eggs in one meal, I think it's best to keep a balance between the yolk and the whites. I personally keep a ratio of about four egg whites to one yolk.

As far as cholesterol is concerned, more and more research suggests that eggs do not raise cholesterol. Eggs contain natural lecithin and, as just mentioned, are one of the highest sources of the natural protein cysteine. Cysteine is crucial for our metabolism and immunity. It's a sensitive protein, though, and is often destroyed when processed. For instance, cysteine is destroyed in most commercial whey protein powders, but whey and colostrum that are processed well does retain it. Eating egg yolks is one of the best ways to supply your body with cysteine. Egg whites are said to be a complete protein, but I feel at least some yolk is necessary to enhance the egg's protein composition and enable you to derive all the benefits of its nutrients. Nature created a white and yellow egg. There are no mistakes in nature, so use both to your advantage. It also tastes better when the whole egg is eaten.

Dairy

Dairy contains a wide variety of tastes, textures, and aromas. Dominant tastes are salty, sour, sweet, pungent, smoked. Textures are smooth, creamy, buttery, milky, oily, soft, hard, chunky, and chewy.

Dairy is a very good whole source of complete protein, and often tastes great. Try to buy organic dairy products. The best sources of dairy protein, and those I highly recommend, are minimally processed fresh, white nonfat or low-fat cheeses like farmer, ricotta, and cottage cheese, and plain yogurt and kefir. Consuming high-fat dairy is not so great, unless it's a raw milk product. Dairy products that are made from raw, organic, non-homogenized and non-pasteurized milk are thought to be the best, but are almost impossible to find due to current governmental regulations.

It's also okay to indulge in aged cheeses, such as a chunk of

Parmesan as an appetizer. Like wine, Parmesan has most of the tastes within it.

Goat, sheep, and buffalo cheeses and yogurt have unique tastes and aromas. They can be great alternatives to cow milk products. Generally speaking, goat, sheep and buffalo dairy products are less allergenic than cow milk products.

If you're not allergic to dairy, that's wonderful, but never take this for granted because if you overeat it you may become sensitive or allergic. So rotate your dairy and don't eat it every day.

Whey Protein

Whey is one of the best sources of protein. If processed right, it's a wonderful protein powder, and a great alternative to other protein foods. I believe when taken on an empty stomach, whey powders will nourish your digestive tract, muscles, and also nourish your brain.

Whey is great to have as a recovery food after a workout, as a light meal during the Undereating Phase, or as a dessert. I don't think whey should be part of the main meal itself since it's a processed powder, and doesn't contain the combination of tastes, aromas, and different textures that whole foods do. And, as mentioned before, you need to experience the array of tastes, textures, and aromas to be truly satisfied. You should eat real food for the main meal and enjoy it. Whey is dairy, so some people are sensitive to it. Monitor yourself.

Warrior Growth Serum and Warrior Milk

Warrior Growth Serum is a proprietary blend of air-dried organic colostrum with other essential nutrients. It's high in immuno-supportive proteins, growth factors, and lactoferin, all of which are essential for full recuperation, tissue repair, muscle building, and overall immunity.

Warrior Milk is a proprietary blend of high-quality dairy protein. It's designed to supply the optimum daily requirement of undenatured protein, meant to provide maximum potential for anabolic protein utilization. More on this can be found in the "Warrior Nutritional Supplements" chapter.

Legumes, Beans, and Peas— the Gladiator Protein

I highly recommend consuming beans and peas, not just because of the fiber and IP6, but also because they're a very good source of protein that's balanced well with complex carbohydrates. And they taste pretty good, too.

The most accessible IP6 is generally found in legumes, beans, and especially peas. A research study conducted on Finnish people found that although they consume one-third as much fiber as the Swedish, they have much less cancer, especially colon cancer, than Swedish people. Researchers believe that this can be attributed to the fact that in Finland the main source of fiber comes from legumes and peas, with their abundant IP6.

Beans contain a high natural source of the protein L-DOPA, which boosts dopamine (a major neurotransmitter) in your brain. Dopamine plays an important role in regulating testosterone and virility. Ancient Romans were aware of the aphrodisiac effects of beans. For thousands of years, Mediterranean people used beans and peas as a major source of protein.

Peas, lentils, and beans were the main source of protein for Greek and Roman civilians and the Roman legions. Beans were also the main source of protein for the gladiators. Warriors hated feeling bloated, so were very careful when selecting beans and with cooking methods. Even given the high consumption of beans at that time, people were ambiguous about them. The full story is very intriguing. I discuss it at greater length in chapter 9, "Lessons from History."

Cooking Protein

History has taught us how to best prepare beef, fish, and fowl.

Ancient Romans cooked protein foods in broth. They often mixed fish or meat with veggies, grain and beans all together in one pot.

The popular practice today of barbecuing or grilling meat, which caramelizes or burns its surface, denatures the protein and creates toxins that are widely believed to be carcinogenic. Any protein can be denatured. Some processing and cooking methods are better, some worse. The "Warrior Meals and Recipes" discusses how to prepare protein meals.

Rotating Protein to Avoid Sensitivities and Allergies

Rotating and varying protein works best. Try not to eat the same group of protein foods on an everyday basis. If you do, you may already be sensitive or allergic to it.

Eggs, for instance, are considered to be one of the most allergenic foods. I personally have never had a problem with eggs, but I don't consume them too often. I have eggs no more than two days per week, and generally rotate chicken, red meat, and fish every other day. I've never had a reaction to chicken or meat either, but everyone is different, so experiment to see what works best for you.

Oils

Oils and fats have a variety of tastes, textures, aromas, and colors. In general, oils add richness to meals as well as a smooth, oily texture.

- **Fat is Essential**
- **Essential Fatty Acids—Yes**
- **Monounsaturated Oils—Yes**
- **Hydrogenated, Partially Hydrogenated Oils—No**
- **Butter—Yes**

- **Margarine—No**
- **Cocoa Butter and Chocolate—Yes**

Essential Fatty Acids

Essential fatty acids (EFA) are the most important oils. Since our bodies cannot produce them, we have to ingest them. They should be part of your main meal. These oils belong to the "living foods" group.

There are some great organic essential fatty acid oils available in the United States, and they can be found in the refrigerated section of health food and vitamin stores. Ideally, your diet should either contain a ratio of 1:1 or 2:1 Omega 3 to Omega 6. Many people suffer from an Omega 3 deficiency. This essential fatty acid appears only in fatty fishes such as salmon, tuna, mackerel, and sardines; and plant sources like flaxseeds, hemp, walnuts, and in small amounts, soy. For those who don't consume enough Omega 3 rich foods, supplementation is necessary (preferably in the form of flaxseed oil, in which Omega 3 is higher than Omega 6).

Omega 6 is abundant in many foods such as grains, nuts, seeds, animal protein, dairy and eggs. Primrose and borage oils are good sources of Omega 6 GLA. GLA is an Omega 6 derivative, a building block for prostaglandins, which regulates blood pressure, inflammation and pain.

Essential fatty acids are best to have with protein and unsweetened carbohydrate meals. Never heat these oils. Fresh flaxseed oil, an Omega 3, has a pleasant nutty taste. Hemp oil contains both Omega 3 and 6 and is very aromatic. Primrose Oil, which is high in Omega 6 GLA, has a light neutral taste.

Essential fatty acids should be carefully processed and handled. Check the expiration date before purchasing and keep them refrigerated. As mentioned, use your senses. Smell oils before you use them. If they have a paint-like smell, it's time to throw them away. Taste them too. You should enjoy these oils. If they don't taste good to you, don't use them. As mentioned, EFA deficiencies, especially of Omega 3, may create serious metabolic problems, including insulin insensitivity.

I know it may sound bizarre, but on the Warrior Diet, healthy fats are unlimited. Use your instinct and trial and error to determine how much oil you want. I generally recommend using between 1–3 tablespoons per day.

Monounsaturated Oils

Monounsaturated oils are generally considered to be the safest oils since they don't oxidize so quickly in the body, and are less sensitive to light and heat. In their raw state, these oils have pleasant natural aromas and are wonderful additions to meals, especially to dry or grainy foods. Olive oil is the least sensitive to light and heat, and so is the best monounsaturated oil to use when cooking. It's also great for dressings and to flavor foods. Use cold pressed extra virgin olive oil to obtain maximum nutritional value.

Avocadoes and almonds contain monounsaturated oils. I highly suggest that you consume them as whole foods. The naturally occurring oil in avocados is in its most biologically potent state when derived from the raw, fresh fruit. The same holds true for almonds. Processing them into oils may take away much of their live properties, especially the enzymes. When consumed in their raw state, avocadoes and almonds are alkalizing and rich in lipase (the enzyme that breaks fat). Loading your body with lipase may also help against obesity and may slow the aging process.

Polyunsaturated Oils

Despite what many health practitioners say, people should be concerned about using polyunsaturated oils/fatty acids such as canola, sunflower, safflower, and corn oil. Most of them don't have enough Omega 3 essential fatty acids and can be destroyed very quickly when heated, exposed to air, etc. High consumption of these oils may lead to an imbalance of essential fatty acids, and a deficiency of Omega 3 may eventually lead to serious metabolic problems.

Hydrogenated and Saturated Oils

These oils have a solid texture at room temperatures. They contain different tastes and aromas. When added to meals they usually enrich flavors, and add a smooth oily texture.

I think it's best to stay away from hydrogenated oils like margarine or processed oils that are found in many commercial foods. Tropical oils like palm or coconut oil are okay as long as they're raw and unprocessed. Regarding butter, while I don't recommend using it extensively, it's okay to have once in a while. Butter is high in saturated fatty acid, however, it does contain a balanced ratio (1:1) of Omega 6 to Omega 3 essential fatty acid, and is rich in vitamins A and E. Butter is preferable to margarine.

Saturated oils are more stable than polyunsaturated oils, so there's less risk of them becoming rancid.

The worst oils to consume are transfatty acids. These are abundant in margarine, hydrogenated oils, and many processed foods. However, some saturated oils— those rich in stearic acid— may actually be good for you. It is believed that chocolate might indeed be an aphrodisiac, and cocoa butter, which is high in stearic acid, may naturally convert in the body to monounsaturated fatty acids, which have a neutral-to-lowering effect on cholesterol. So, in addition to other surprises, the Warrior Diet allows you to indulge in—yes—chocolate, following protein meals, preferably dark chocolate.

Nuts and Seeds

Nuts and seeds have different tastes, textures, and aromas. They add a crunchy texture and different nutty aromas and flavors to meals.

Nuts

A variety of nuts are allowed and suggested on the Warrior Diet. Raw and lightly roasted nuts are both good, but raw nuts are better since they nourish you with healthy oil and live enzymes, which the roasting process may destroy. Lipase (the enzyme that breaks fat) is abundant in raw nuts and seeds. As mentioned before, lipase is essential for your fat metabolism. Eating raw, high-fat foods such as nuts and seeds is a natural way to load your body with lipase.

The Warrior Rule of Nuts—Nutty Meals

On the Warrior Diet you can actually consume as many raw nuts as you'd like, and still not gain weight. Just follow this rule: Do not consume nuts with grain carbohydrates. Nuts work very well with a small amount of protein and with an abundant amount of veggies. You can basically live on nuts and veggies, eat as much as you want of them, and still not gain weight. Actually I believe you're going to lose some weight. Try this for a couple of days and see for yourself. Just make sure you chew them extremely well to ensure maximum digestibility. For a "nut-and-veggie" diet, the best nuts are almonds. An almond-veggie diet will give you a nice body odor, almost like a vanilla-almond scent. Sounds too good to be true? Well, that's the way life should be.

Almonds

Almonds are highly recommended. They are a great source of proteins, minerals, vitamins, monounsaturated fats, and an excellent natural source of zinc. Almonds have long been considered to be an aphrodisiac food. Ancient Hindus, Hebrews, and Romans saw the almond as a symbol of female, as well as male, genitals. I truly believe that almonds are an aphrodisiac food, partly because of their mineral composition, partly because of their fat content, and partly due to their alkalizing effect. Edgar Cayce, among other holistic healers, considered almonds to possess anticancerous properties. It's interesting to note that almonds are believed to be a homeopathic remedy since they contain a minuscule amount of cyanide, which some say works like a natural chemotherapy agent in the body that destroys sick cells and tumors.

Almonds ideally should be eaten raw. In their raw state they're the only nut that alkalizes your body. It is okay, however, to occasionally eat lightly roasted almonds. They're still good for you and some prefer their taste. It's best to eat roasted almonds soon after you roast them to avoid rancidity.

Peanuts

Peanuts aren't really nuts. They belong to the legume family.

According to Dr. Peter D'Adamo, author of Eat Right for Your Type, research shows that peanuts have anticancerous properties, especially the red skin around them. Just make sure you're not allergic to them! I personally like to eat peanuts in moderation because over consumption is acidic and for some this will be a problem, and may make them harder to digest. Also, peanuts may contain some mold toxins, which is believed to be cancerous.

On a positive note, peanuts are high in protein and contain essential fatty acids (mainly Omega 6). The oil in peanuts is relatively stable, which is why peanuts, their butter, and oils are used so often throughout the world in various dishes, sauces, and even protein bars.

Cashews

Cashews are one of the least allergenic nuts. They are naturally high in iron. If you like them raw, that's the best. To be on the safe side, seek out organic cashews. Note: Most cashews come from India, and go through a fumigating process before they can be exported. So, it's unlikely that you'll find unprocessed raw cashews.

Walnuts

Walnuts are one of the most nutritious nuts and they contain Omega 3 essential fatty acid. Since their fat content is very high, you shouldn't eat more than a handful or two at any one time. To avoid indigestion, eat walnuts in moderation.

Pine Nuts

Pine nuts do not contain the ideal fat, but are a very good supplemental nut because of their antioxidant properties. Ancient Romans and Greeks used them often as a supplemental food, adding them mainly to grains to enhance taste and density. Pine nuts continue to be used in this way today, particularly in the Mediterranean.

Pistachios

One of the biggest advantages of the pistachio, besides the fact that it tastes so good, is that it's one of the least allergenic nuts. Very few people have reactions to pistachios, even if they react to all other nuts. Pistachios were popular all throughout the Roman Empire, especially in the Middle East and North Africa, and remain popular in many regions of the world today.

Thoughts on Salted Nuts

Although they're allowed, I think salted nuts aren't always the best idea, because salty means processed, which means containing less natural properties. Salted, roasted nuts can, however, accelerate satiety simply because they'll make you thirsty sooner than unsalted nuts, and some people prefer their taste.

Seeds

Seeds belong to the same high-fat food group as nuts. They are highly nutritious. To avoid indigestion, don't consume too many seeds at any one time; a half handful will do. I think of seeds as a supplemental food. It's best to eat them either alone as a snack, or with protein meals.

Seeds contain a higher content of fat than nuts. Sesame, pumpkin, and sunflower seeds are all good sources of oils, flavones, and other components that support and maintain optimum health. Pumpkin seeds, for example, are one of the highest natural sources of zinc. Seeds, such as pumpkin and sunflower, are thought to help protect your hormonal system and are considered to be an aphrodisiac food. Sunflower seeds are very sensitive to light and so ideally should be kept in a dark container to avoid rancidity. Seeds are rich in plant sterols and sterolines, which are oil substances that are believed to support the hormonal system and have cholesterol-lowering properties.

My thoughts on raw versus roasted seeds is the same as those for nuts. Both are good, but raw is always better.

Lecithin

Lecithin is a natural source of phospholipids, which are the building blocks of cell membranes. Lecithin has a nutty, buttery taste. Besides being a good source of phospholipids, it's also high in choline, and inositol, which are building blocks for brain neurotransmitters.

Lecithin is a natural emulsifier, helping the liver to metabolize triglicerides. Thus, lecithin is a wonderful aid for liver detoxification and fat metabolism.

I usually put a tablespoon or two on top of my protein meals just before eating.

Carbohydrates

Carbohydrates display different tastes, with sweet or starchy being most dominant. They have different aromas and textures: light, heavy, grainy, smooth, chewy, creamy and crunchy.

Complex and Simple Carbs

Most people know that there are two kinds of carbohydrates, complex and simple. Consuming complex carbohydrates, whole grains, is usually much more beneficial than consuming simple carbohydrates, but not always. Sometimes, simple natural carbohydrate-rich foods, such as papaya or pineapple, can be the best complement to a meal. Adding more flavors and textures is partly why, but the main reason is that meat is usually digested more easily when eaten with certain fruits. Combining meat with fruit is a very old tradition. Hunter-gatherers hunted meat and also gathered berries, and often ate them together. In tropical areas people often marinate meats with papaya or pineapple juices. The protease enzymes found in these tropical fruits predigests the meat and makes it softer and more tender.

Whole grains are best to eat when they're fully cooked. Soaking, rinsing, and cooking removes toxins, and makes the fiber soft and more edible.

Pleasure, Satiety and Relaxation

Carbohydrates create satiety since they naturally boost serotonin production in your brain. Serotonin is a protein neurotransmitter that binds to the pleasure receptors in certain areas in your brain. Once this happens, you may feel calmer, happier, more satisfied, and be able to sleep better since serotonin is also a building block for the hormone melatonin.

Here are some reasons why it's good to eat carbohydrates as the last component of your meal:

1. Control Your Insulin

We don't want to unnecessarily boost too much insulin.

It's better to consume a meal with the lowest glycemic index. The higher the glycemic index is, the more pressure is placed on your body to produce insulin. When veggies are eaten first, followed by protein and fat, the glycemic index of any carb that is consumed afterwards is automatically reduced.

2. Follow the First Rule of Eating

Carbs generally have more dominant, aggressive tastes than veggies or protein, and the more processed they are, the more aggressive they become. Since the first rule of eating is to begin with subtle tastes and move to the more aggressive, carbohydrates should in general be eaten last. You can skip carbs entirely if you reach full satiety after eating the veggies and protein part of the meal. You don't have to eat carbs every day. It's also good to rotate between relatively low and relatively moderate carb days.

3. Lose Body Fat

If you want to lose body fat, have carbohydrates as the last component of your meal (after protein). This method naturally minimizes the amount of carbs that you eat without feeling deprived. The fewer carbs you ingest the more fat you burn.

Choosing Carbohydrates— What Are The Best Carbs To Eat?

Plants and Roots

The safest sources of carbohydrates (meaning the least reactive, and with minimal insulin fluctuations) come from plants and roots, like carrots, beets, pumpkin and all the squash family. Potatoes, corn, plantains, and cassava are more starchy and dense, and have a higher glycemic index. Therefore, they're somewhat more reactive with insulin. All these plant foods are rich in vital nutrients, such as minerals, flavones, and fiber, and most of them need to be cooked.

It is my opinion that consuming whole food carbohydrates is the best way to reach satisfaction instinctually. The two factors that help one to reach satiety are the minerals and fiber content that are within these foods. When one eats foods which are high in naturally occurring minerals and fiber, it triggers an instinctive feedback mechanism in the body that recognizes full nourishment and satisfaction. Conversely, eating refined, processed carbohydrate foods, which lack naturally occurring minerals and fiber, leads to feelings of deprivation, and this often expresses itself as compulsive bingeing.

Fruits

Fruits aren't necessarily a good choice of carbs for the main meal. However, fruits are loaded with phytonutrients, vitamins, minerals, and living enzymes in their most potent form. Since the Undereating Phase is based on ingesting live fruits and veggies, with their detoxifying, catabolic, alkalizing quality, I believe that in order to balance the body into more of an acidic, anabolic state, and to reach full satisfaction from your meal, you should minimize fruits during the main meal and instead consume more plants, roots, and grains. There are, however, exceptions. As noted, you can complement high protein meals with berries, tropical fruits, and fermented fruits, which are relatively low in sugar and high in enzymes.

Grains

Next to plants and roots, the best source of carbs comes from grains, such as rice, quinoa, barley, and millet.

Rice

Rice is a highly nutritious grain, and very few people are sensitive to it. Ideally you should develop a taste for whole-grain brown rice, with the fiber. Whole grain rice is rich in B vitamins and rice bran, and high in a complex of vital nutrients, including tocopherols, which are believed to be the most potent form of vitamin E. But, if you'd rather have white rice at times, this is also fine. I sometimes prefer white rice. Let your taste and mood be your guide.

Barley—the Gladiator Grain

An advantage of barley, in addition to its high-protein content, is that barley broth helps detoxify the liver. And, when compared to all grains, it has one of the lowest glycemic indexes. Barley was a major grain and ingredient in bread for both the ancient Romans and Greeks, and a main food of the gladiators. Gladiators were often called "Barley Carriers" in mocking reference to the animals that used to transport barley.

Barley is often used in soups, but can also be eaten as porridge, or as part of a cooked meal, just as you'd serve rice.

Quinoa

Quinoa isn't really a grain; it's actually the fruit of an herb that's grown in the Andes. It's high in protein, and contains all eight essential amino acids plus potassium, iron, and zinc. Quinoa requires only a short cooking time. It has a mild flavor and a fluffy, slightly sticky texture. It's one of the safest grains to ingest.

Millet

Millet is an alkaline grain. Its protein content is higher than that found in wheat, corn, or rice. It's popular in India, Africa, China, and Russia. Millet is the least allergenic of all grains.

Amaranth

Another choice is amaranth. It is high in protein, and is actually a complete protein with a roughly equivalent protein composition to that found in red meat. Like quinoa, amaranth is not really a grain; it's a fruit. There are different ways to eat amaranth, including toasting it so it pops like popcorn. It tastes pretty earthy when prepared other ways. Those who've never eaten it should prepare themselves for something completely different. Some people find its taste to be too strong and aromatic. You've got to try it to determine if you like it. Amaranth, by the way, was the food of the Aztecs and their gods. Amaranth can be found in many forms in most health food stores.

Oats

Oats are also a very good grain. I like oatmeal, but rarely include it as part of my main meal. With meat or fish, I prefer to have plant carbohydrates, rice, or other grains. Meat and rice or meat and potatoes simply works better for me than meat and oatmeal.

I know that most people like to have oatmeal in the morning, but the Warrior Diet does not suggest having carbs during the Undereating Phase (unless you are an extremely physically active person). In the "Warrior Diet Idea" I discuss how you can alternate the Warrior Diet with days of high protein and days of high carbs. You can basically live on oatmeal on high carb days.

I think oatmeal goes very well with certain proteins, like eggs or yogurt. Oatmeal is very high in water-soluble fiber and B vitamins, which are essential for your health.

Wheat and Buckwheat

The least desirable grain is wheat because a lot of people have reactions to it, or are sensitive to the gluten inside. Wheat may also be mildly estrogenic for some people. And it is one of the most acidic grains. The wheat we eat today is not the same as it was in the past, and modern wheat contains a higher percentage of gluten. So be cautious with it. And, be cautious with buckwheat, too.

According to Dr. Peter D'Adamo, author of Eat Right for Your Type, people with blood type O should avoid wheat, and those with blood type B and AB should avoid buckwheat. On a positive note, since buckwheat doesn't belong to the wheat family, it doesn't contain gluten. Buckwheat is also high in complete protein.

You can find gluten free breads, cereals, and pastas in many health food stores.

Sprouted Wheat

Sprouted wheat is different from regular wheat. The sprouting destroys most of the gluten. It's also less acidic than common wheat, and is a good source of enzymes and bran. Sprouted wheat breads are available in health food stores. Check the ingredients to make sure that sprouted wheat is the main ingredient in the flour.

Kamut and Spelt

They belong to the wheat family. Many who eat them experience more or less similar, but usually milder, symptoms than common wheat. These grains can be eaten as porridge or as part of a whole-grain meal. You can also find them in puffed and other dry cereals, and as puffed cakes (like rice cakes).

Dry Cereals

Carbohydrates are generally best to ingest when they're fresh, cooked, warm, and somewhat moist. But, and listen to this (big time), there's an alternative way to eat them. I call it "chewing dry cereal." There are some very good, unsweetened dry cereals on the market today, usually sold in health food stores or the health-food section of supermarkets. The best ones are organic. I like those that are made from puffed rice, corn, or a combination of corn and amaranth, but there's a whole host of other options as well. Companies like Nature's Path, Erewon, and Arrowhead Mills make delicious dry cereals. The ideal time to eat dry cereals is toward the end of the meal, right after protein.

The advantage of dry cereal is that you use a lot of your saliva, which helps pre-digest the food. When you eat wet cereal, you don't chew it as much as when it's dry. The more you chew, the better you're going to digest the food, and I believe the more satiety you'll experience. Dry cereals add a crunchy texture to the meal. If you add essential fatty acids on top of these cereals it will lower the glycemic index, enrich the nutritional value, and might even make them taste better.

If you like eating your cereal with milk, note that you may miss the whole point of chewing dry cereal. However, if you like to add milk, go for skim or low-fat. You can also use grain milk instead. However, most of these contain sugars so use them in moderation. If you're trying to lose body fat, stick to unsweetened dry cereal. Think of it as eating popcorn.

Sweet Meals for "Sweet Teeth"

The carbohydrate stage of the Warrior Diet is one of choice. You're given two choices and must select either a sweet meal or starchy one.

Sweet meals are not the preferred choice. But for those who like to have something sweet for dessert, here's what to do.

Have a high protein meal with veggies (such as zucchini, broccoli, spinach, Swiss chard, string beans, eggplant, or vegetables). Moderate your fat intake on these days as well (fat and sugar aren't an ideal combination; sugar may disturb optimum EFA metabolism). At the end of the meal you can indulge in a sweet dessert. But, try to avoid simple (common processed) sugars, hydrogenated and partially hydrogenated fats. They're always bad for you.

I suggest and explain how to prepare some dessert recipes, such as pumpkin cheesecake and fruit gelatin, which contain minimal carbohydrates, yet taste like a sweet, delicious dessert (see "Warrior Meals and Recipes"). And, as noted earlier, it's okay to eat chocolate at the end of the meal if you want to. Just make sure you treat it as a condiment.

Here's a tip:

Natural sweeteners like raw honey or brown rice syrup can be mixed with protein (like whey powder). It'll add texture, taste, and may stop sugar cravings at the end of your meal. Moreover, especially for athletes, this is a good way to add protein to your diet.

Sample Sweet Meal

First Course—Salad

Main Course—Fish and Eggplant

Dessert—Pumpkin Cheesecake

Starchy Meals

The second choice, which I generally prefer, is to have complex carbohydrates (starches), and no sweet dessert. Remember, even though carbs are unlimited, it's best that they come at the end of the meal; particularly for those whose goal is to lose body fat. If you like to mix carbohydrates with protein, that's okay. As noted earlier, eating carbs alone, without protein or fat accompanying it, often causes over stimulation of insulin, which eventually leads to insulin insensitivity, blood-sugar fluctuations, and fat gain.

Fiber

Fiber contains different textures: pectins, mucilage, and gums are soft and gummy, cellulose and bran are solid, coarse, and crumby.

Having fiber in your diet is critical for your health. Fiber helps keep insulin in balance, feeds healthy gut bacteria, helps prevent constipation, reduces cholesterol, and protects against cancer. Unfortunately, when many people eat fibrous food they become bloated and gassy. Those who find this to be so should monitor themselves and eliminate from their diet those fibers to which they're sensitive. It's not unusual for people to react poorly to one kind of fiber, and better to others. Note that loading your body with enzymes may help digest fibrous foods and alleviate the above side effects.

In my opinion, if you take a high-quality probiotic supplement, you can reduce your fiber consumption somewhat and should still keep your digestion and elimination systems intact. More on this is in the "Warrior Nutritional Supplements."

Fermented Foods

Fermented foods contain a variety of tastes, textures, and aromas. They enhance the composition of the meal and thus fall within the second rule of eating. The dominant taste of fermented food is sour. Textures and aromas vary according to the food.

Naturally fermented foods are high in lactic-acid producing bacteria. This helps the digestive process and optimizes metabolism.

Fermented foods (that when naturally fermented are good sources of beneficial bacteria) include:

Pickles	Apple Cider Vinegar
Olives	Yogurt (preferably plain)
Sauerkraut	Kefir (preferably plain)
Miso Soup	

Fermentation helps protect food from spoiling. Warriors used to carry fermented foods with them in tough weather, like desert climates, for a long time. The lactic-acid producing bacteria within naturally fermented foods is what prevents spoilage; and this good bacterium destroys pathogenic bacteria. In fact, consumption of naturally fermented foods is also one of the best ways to naturally help rid yourself of yeast infections, which affect much of the western population today. Yeast infections are the result of a chronic imbalance of gut flora, and are usually caused by the continual consumption of sugar, overly processed and junk foods, and taking antibiotics. Naturally fermented foods are also a wonderful aid in the production of certain B vitamins as well as Vitamin D.

Moreover, the lactic acid-forming bacteria within fermented foods complete the final digestion of amino acids, thereby creating better protein efficiency. Traditionally, fermented food accompanied high protein meals. This fact is extremely important for athletes who generally consume much more protein than the general population. Lactic acid-producing bacteria balances the pH in the colon, which may protect against bacterial infections and cancer.

The Japanese traditionally pickle eggplants, a variety of exotic vegetables, roots, and even fruits. In India, mangoes and papayas are pickled, and used as a chutney relish to eat with meat. Mediterranean food is enriched with pickles, olives, and sauerkraut. Indonesian food is also full of relishes and fermented foods. Ancient Romans used to pickle almost anything, including fish and dairy. Let me note here that not every sour food is naturally fermented. Real fermentation requires lactic acid-producing bacteria as a natural catalyst.

Fermented foods can be eaten at any stage of the meal. It's preferable to eat them before or with protein. You should monitor the amount of fermented food that you consume. Start with small amounts and increase gradually in order to avoid unpleasant symptoms, like bloating.

Fermentation destroys sugar by converting it to lactic acid. For those who are lactose-intolerant, eating fermented dairy, such as plain yogurt or kefir, may be of benefit, because under fermentation most of the lactose sugar is destroyed.

Apple Cider Vinegar

Apple cider vinegar is a good source of food enzymes and minerals, and so could be a good live supplement for your digestion and overall health. I'm not, however, a big fan of vinegar in general because it also feeds bad bacteria and may cause yeast. And, vinegar increases acidity sometimes in an uncontrolled manner. If your diet is too alkaline, vinegar (in moderation) could be helpful. It has a balancing factor. But if you're too acidic, stay away from all vinegars.

Wine

Wine contains most of the tastes (with a dominance of sour, sweet, dry, and pungent), different aromas, and a smooth texture. Wine is a live fermented food. When you sense its taste, your brain already starts to reach a level of satiety.

Wine is good for digestion since it contains many enzymes. It can also help combat free radicals, and studies have shown that the flavones in red wine may protect against heart attacks. Drinking wine in moderation may help keep us healthy.

A lot of people drink a glass of wine just before, or with, their dinner. This is acceptable on the Warrior Diet, as I believe, speaking generally, that drinking a glass of good wine just before, or with, dinner enriches a meal.

Wine can have some negative side effects, including:

- It may tax the liver
- The alcohol content may have an estrogenic effect on some people's bodies
- Some people are sensitive to the sulfites that are in most wines and experience allergic reactions to sulfites
- Drinking wine may exacerbate overacidity in those who already suffer from it
- If you suffer from toxicity, drinking alcohol will make this worse
- Pregnant women should avoid all alcohol

The Acid-Base Balancing Factor

In addition to balancing tastes, textures, aromas and temperatures, it's important to reach a healthy acid-base balance of your meal in order to keep the second rule of eating intact.

You can control your acid-alkaline balance on the Warrior Diet without compromising the quality of food or the amount you eat. Since the Undereating Phase is based on consumption of living foods like fruits, vegetables, and their freshly prepared juices, which are potent alkalizers, you actually pre-potentiate your body's pH and your enzyme pool for the Overeating Phase, which is based on more acid-forming foods, such as meats and certain grains.

Consuming a lot of vegetables with the main meal, in addition to the advantages mentioned earlier, is also alkalizing. Regarding grains, some are less acidic. For example, millet is an alkalizing grain; quinoa, too. All the grains that belong to the wheat family are more acidic.

People Whose System Is Too Alkaline

Those people whose systems are too alkaline can use vinegar (rice vinegar or organic apple cider vinegar are good choices) in order to instantly acidify the overalkaline system. Eating high protein meals naturally acidifies the body. All animal proteins (besides raw milk) are acid-forming foods.

People Who Suffer From Overacidity

Those who suffer from overacidity, which is the case for the majority of people, should consume more live and cooked veggies, since they are alkalizing, and avoid all vinegars. I also recommend consuming foods that are high in minerals, such as miso, which is made from nonpasteurized, fermented soybeans. Miso is a wonderful alkalizer that's rich in minerals and organic sodium. It can be consumed as a soup or as a sauce. Another way to instantly alkalize the body is supplementing with good quality highly ionized minerals, such as coral-derived minerals. (For more on this, go to the "Warrior Diet Nutritional Supplements" chapter.)

Glycemic Index

The glycemic index (GI) shows how much insulin your body secretes when a food or beverage is introduced into your blood. Although this sounds simple, it's actually quite confusing. For instance, the same food can have a different GI depending on how it's cooked. Pasta al dente (pasta that's cooked for a shorter time, and so remains slightly hard), has a lower glycemic index than well-cooked soft pasta. Baked potatoes have a higher glycemic index than mashed potatoes because of a difference in the macrostructure of the carbohydrate.

When you add butter, milk, monounsaturated oil, or essential fatty acids to food, it usually lowers the GI. So, if you eat a baked potato with oil, for instance, it has a lower glycemic index than eating a plain baked potato. Fiber slows carbohydrate absorption and therefore may help reduce the glycemic index of the carbs ingested. Whole grains have a lower glycemic index than refined grains.

Even though many people consider the glycemic index as the parameter for selecting carbs, I don't believe that the GI is always as critical a factor as it's believed to be. Fructose, for example, has a lower GI than white rice. But, in my opinion, commercial fructose, which appears in many commercial foods, processed foods, and health bars, is one of the most dangerous and destructive sources of carbs. White rice, with its higher GI, is a far superior choice. Fruit juices and certain vegetable juices (like carrot juice) have a relatively high GI, but since they come from natural, live (raw) foods (I'm referring to juices that are freshly squeezed) the body can usually handle them very well. Freshly prepared juices contain digestive enzymes that help metabolize naturally occurring sugars into energy. Live (raw) natural fruits and vegetables also load the body with essential nutrients that support overall metabolism. So, even though fruits and certain veggies have a relatively high GI, it's not something to worry about, unless you are diabetic or hypoglycemic.

The exception is grapes. They're high in glucose which causes rapid rises in blood sugar and therefore may trigger undesirable insulin spikes. As noted, grapes should be avoided or eaten in moderation during the day. I sometimes have grapes for dessert after a high protein evening meal.

Salt Restriction

I question the effectiveness of salt restriction. When you restrict sodium, in the beginning you might lose some water weight, but if you reintroduce it, you may suffer from water retention. The reason for this is that sodium restriction triggers a spike in the hormone aldosterone (one of the adrenocortex hormones secreted by the adrenal glands, which works to preserve sodium inside the tissue cells), and this process creates water retention. As long as you keep sodium intake fairly consistent and in a normal ratio (which, of course, should be slightly higher in warmer weather, and after extensive aerobic activity), you won't over-secrete this hormone, or trigger what I call the "aldosterone syndrome."

Healthy people who routinely consume sodium generally don't experience ill effects by increasing it somewhat. It's those who restrict sodium consumption and then suddenly increase it who usually suffer from water retention. This is unfortunately what happens to many body builders. During the competitive season, when sodium is restricted, they look leaner, but sometimes hours after the first meal that's no longer sodium-restricted—boom—they can blow up like a balloon.

Keeping The Sodium Pump Intact

Balancing sodium intake has a lot to do with the ratio of sodium to potassium and magnesium. Natural foods, like fruits and veggies, whole grains, and roots, have a high ratio of potassium to sodium (up to 200:1). Unfortunately, the typical American overly processed diet has an opposite ratio in which sodium is higher than potassium. To say this simply, in order to regulate your sodium intake, make sure that you balance your potassium-to-sodium ratio. Ideally, your potassium intake should be higher than your sodium intake. Potassium is antagonistic to sodium.

It drives excessive sodium out of the cells, and thus keeps your sodium-potassium pump intact, helping protect against water retention and high blood pressure.

The best salts to consume are sea salts. My favorites are those that come from the Dead Sea.

Iodized salt is a fair option for those who suffer from an iodine deficiency. However, the best sources of organic iodine come from fish, seafood and sea vegetables.

Note: This advice relates to healthy people. Those who suffer from high or low blood pressure, arthritis, or heart problems should first consult their physician.

The Most Allergenic Foods

The most allergenic foods are dairy products, eggs, wheat, corn, soy, peanuts, and sugar--and all the foods made with them. There are many other foods that people are allergic to as well, including shellfish, chocolate, yeast, potatoes, aspartame, citrus fruits, coffee, chamomile tea, MSG, additives, and a host of others. Monitor yourself. Those who feel sensitivity to certain foods should avoid them and consider seeing an allergist. In any case, it's always a wise idea to rotate all the foods you consume to avoid developing sensitivities and allergies.

What is Not Allowed on the Warrior Diet

Almost everything is allowed on the Warrior Diet, but there are a few exceptions:

• Refined Sugar
• Refined, Processed Pastries

These are not allowed on the Warrior Diet. Combining starch with excessive sugar does not work, never has, and it never will. I feel that if the sugar content per 2 oz. serving of a starchy treat is less than 2 grams, then it's okay. I don't recommend more than this because it may place unnecessary pressure on your pancreatic system to rapidly increase insulin production. You should also read the ingredients to check the quality of the leavening, as well as the chemicals and preservatives used in baked products. If they contain aluminum-based leavening, artificial food coloring, nitrites, sulfites, hydrogenated or partially hydrogenated oils, or simple sugars, stay away from these pastries, cookies, and candies. If you choose to consume them, fine, but when you do, you're not following the Warrior Diet.

END NOTE:

If you're just completing this chapter and still find the information confusing or a bit overwhelming, just remember to follow the Warrior Diet's Three Rules of Eating. This is a great way to start.

Rule #1: Always start with subtle tasting foods and move to the more aggressive foods.

Rule #2: Include as many tastes, textures, colors, and aromas as possible in your main meal.

Rule #3: Stop eating when you feel much more thirsty than hungry.

By practicing this diet, you'll gradually remember more of the details, which will help you to define and reach your goals. This is a very personal and creative diet. As long as you follow the above rules, you'll soon find your own unique diet, the one that works best for you. Trust your instincts.

The Warrior Diet Daily Food Cycle: When and What to Eat and Drink

This is for all those people who say to me, "Ori, just tell me what I can eat during the day and what I can eat at night."

- **Eat raw fruits and vegetables during the day; all food groups at night.**

- **Drink plenty of clean, pure water throughout the day.**

Mornings through Noon:
- Water—drink at least one glass of water upon awakening, preferably two (either plain, or with a lemon or orange wedge)
- Coffee or tea
- Fruits—fresh, raw fruits
- Juices—freshly prepared from raw vegetables or fruits. I mean really fresh, those made to order in a blender or juicer, not pre-prepared or bottled juices

Noon through end of day:
- Coffee or tea
- Fruits—fresh, raw fruits
- Juices—freshly prepared from raw vegetables (such as carrot, beet, parsley juice) or raw fruits (such as oranges, grapefruits, strawberries, blueberries)
- Miso soup

During the adaptation period, and days that you feel deprived:

- Green salad, with little or no dressing
- Protein—Warrior Growth Serum would be the protein of choice during the day
- Or you can opt for lean protein (no more than 6 oz.), such as: sashimi, eggs, chicken breast, turkey breast, fish, shellfish, plain yogurt or kefir (low-fat or nonfat), cottage cheese, or whey protein. Don't mix proteins; have only one per day
- Raw nuts: A handful of raw nuts, preferably almonds, instead of lean protein

- **The Warrior Diet is based on the principle of eating one large meal per day, preferably at night. During this meal you can eat as much as you want.**

Evenings:

Eat as much as you want from all the food groups (protein, fat, and carbohydrates), as long as you follow the Warrior Diet rules of eating:

1. Start with *leafy green vegetables* (such as romaine lettuce red leaf lettuce, arugula, parsley, endives)

2. Continue with *protein* (such as chicken breast, turkey breast, fish, shellfish, veal scaloppini, sirloin steak, filet mignon, eggs, cottage cheese), *cooked vegetables* (such as broccoli, cauliflower, zucchini, carrots, squash, mushrooms, eggplant, beet greens, kale, collard greens), and *fat* (such as essential fatty acid (EFA) oils, olive oil, almonds, avocado, butter)

3. Finish with *carbohydrates* (such as rice, potatoes, corn, yams, quinoa, barley)

4. Stop eating when you feel much more thirsty than hungry

Before and after your workout:

Before:
Water
Coffee or tea
Warrior Growth Serum

After:
1 liter of water, during and after
Warrior Live Minerals
Warrior Growth Serum
Warrior Milk

Extremely Active People

For professional athletes and others who engage in intense vigorous physical activities during the day, and burn thousands of calories, it may be necessary to consume more food during the day to satisfy high-calorie demands, and to spare muscle breakdown. In these circumstances, it's okay to have a light carbohydrate meal during the day (such as oatmeal and eggs, rice 'n' eggs, rice soup, or barley soup). However, if your goal is to lose body fat, minimize the amount of carbohydrates during the day, and have a light protein meal, preferably Warrior Growth Serum or Warrior Milk.

The Warrior Diet—A Sample Day

Upon Awakening:
2 cups of water
Vitamin C—1000mg
Grape Seed Extract—200mg
Milk Thistle (standardized)— 175mg
Probiotics—2–5 capsules
Warriorzyme—4 capsules
Warrior Minerals—2 capsules
Ginkgo Biloba (standardized)—60mg
Coffee—black, from freshly ground beans

Morning Shake

Small grapefruit juice
Warrior Growth Serum—10–15g

Noon

Medium size juice—carrot, beat, and ginger
Korean Ginseng (standardized)—200mg

Early Afternoon

A bowl of berries

Late Afternoon

Warrior Growth Serum—20–30g
Coffee—black or espresso with milk foam

Early Evening: Workout

During and after the workout
1–1.5 lt. water
Multivitamin
Warrior Minerals—4 capsules
Vitamin C—1000mg
Warriorzyme—4 capsules
Recovery meal: Warrior Milk—30–50g

Evening: Main Meal

Mixed green salad (you can add tomatoes, onions, and olive oil)
Curry chicken in spicy tomato broth
EFA oil, lecithin
Steamed broccoli, zucchini, and carrots
(Eat as much as you wan t from all the above)

If you are fully satisfied or much more thirsty than hungry, stop eating. If you are still hungry, finish with brown rice tapioca with EFA or lecithin.

Alternatively, finish with a Warrior Diet Dessert like Pumpkin Cheesecake.
Green tea with ginger, slightly sweetened with maple syrup.

Late Night Shake

Warrior Growth Serum or Warrior Milk

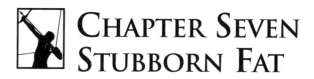

CHAPTER SEVEN
STUBBORN FAT

Stubborn fat is a major problem for many people today. It doesn't matter if they are trying to get rid of it through various diets or different exercise routines—the fact is, this fat remains and seems impossible to remove. That's why it's called stubborn fat. I'm not aware of any diet that seriously addresses this problem.

Liposuction is the most popular method today of removing stubborn fat. Liposuction sucks out fat tissues through surgery. This can be dangerous, or even fatal, and it often doesn't solve the problem. Such extreme measures just show how desperate people are. This is a multimillion-dollar industry today.

There are natural, noninvasive ways to remove stubborn fat. To understand how to deal with this problem, let me explain:

1. What stubborn fat is
2. Why we have it
3. How to prevent it
4. If you have it, how to get rid of it

What is Stubborn Fat?

Stubborn fat is a slow-metabolized adipose (fat) tissue. To burn fat, a natural hormonal process has to take place. When a fat-burning process is activated, the adrenal hormones (adrenaline and noradrenaline) bind to special receptors in the fat tissues. There are two major groups of receptors in the fat tissues, alpha and beta. The beta-receptors are the more active ones, which respond to the adrenal hormones. Fat burning occurs when the adrenal hormones activate the beta-receptors in the fat cells. If these receptors are not activated, no fat will burn off.

Stubborn fat has a lower ratio of beta-receptors to alpha-receptors. As a result, it's metabolized slowly and does not respond to the adrenal hormones. To make matters worse, stubborn fat has more estrogen receptors in the tissues. Estrogen (the female hormone), once bound to the receptors, causes even more fat gain.

There's much more to it, but I don't want to make this very complicated and too scientific. So for now, let's just say that stubborn fat presents three major problems:

1. It doesn't have a high enough ratio of beta-receptors to alpha-receptors, so doesn't respond to adrenal fat-burning stimulation.

2. It has more estrogen receptors, which accelerates fat gain.

And, on top of all this,

3. Stubborn fat doesn't have a healthy blood circulation. These slowly metabolized fat tissues have fewer blood vessels than a normal fat tissue, and consequently it makes this fat slower to metabolize and, therefore, more stubborn or difficult to remove.

What Causes Stubborn Fat?

There are many reasons for having stubborn fat. Both men and women may suffer from it as a result of maintaining an unhealthy diet, from the liver's inability to break down and detoxify estrogenic derivatives, or due to sensitivity to certain foods or chemicals within foods. Fat gain has also been associated with insulin insensitivity and over-consumption of carbohydrates. Consuming too many carbohydrates—especially sugar and overly-processed, refined carbs—places pressure on the pancreas to overproduce insulin in order to lower blood sugar levels.

Hyperinsulinemia causes insulin insensitivity. When this happens, the body converts these extra carbohydrates into triglycerides and fat.

Deficiencies in certain nutrients, vitamins, and minerals—such as B vitamins, chromium, magnesium, zinc, and omega 3 essential fatty acid (alpha-linolenic acid)—may also cause insulin insensitivity and compromise fat metabolism in cellular mitochondria (compounds in the cells that are responsible for energy production and fat burning).

Stubborn fat can be linked to protein deficiencies as well. Vegetarians and vegans are more likely to suffer from protein deficiencies, and especially to the essential amino acid lysine. Lysine, abundant in animal proteins but less so in grains, converts in our bodies to L-carnitine. Carnitine is an amino acid essential for the fat-burning process. Carnitine appears only in animal foods, especially red meat. Without enough carnitine and carnitine-related enzymes in your system, the ability to burn fat is severely compromised.

Stubborn fat can be an age-related problem for men. The older men get, the more testosterone is converted into estrogen—this process is called aromatization. The older you get, the more the aromatase enzyme is active. Fat tissues produce aromatase enzymes and therefore accelerate the action which converts testosterone into estrogen. There are natural ways that may block this process. We'll discuss them soon.

Women usually suffer from age-related stubborn fat around their hips, thighs, and butt. Some women have stubborn-fat tissues around their upper arms or entire legs. Age-related stubborn fat for women may be the result of hormonal fluctuations, or an increase in estrogen receptors in the tissues. Moreover, age-related insulin insensitivity, chronic stress, liver congestion, low thyroid, vascular permeability, and exhausted adrenals may all make the syndrome even worse for both men and women.

How to Prevent Stubborn Fat

There are several things you can do to avoid stubborn fat:

1. Stay away from crash diets or diets that make you lose fat and gain it again. Second-generation fat is more stubborn than the first. The more you fluctuate with your weight, the more stubborn fat you may gain.

2. Avoid consuming foods that you may be sensitive or allergic to. Some people react to certain foods, such as wheat, dairy, or soy. If you suspect this may be the case, get yourself checked for food sensitivities.

3. Eat as much organic food as possible, thereby avoiding many estrogenic substances that are in our food supply, like petroleum and other chemically based fertilizers, pesticides, and herbicides (found in nonorganic produce), and hormones, which are found in nonorganic meats, poultry, dairy and eggs.

4. Drink pure, filtered water. Don't drink or cook with tap water that is unfiltered.

5. If the food or liquid smells like plastic, stay away from it.

6. Minimize your alcohol consumption. Excessive alcohol may compromise your liver's ability to break down and detoxify estrogenic derivatives. When not broken down and detoxified, these estrogenic toxins penetrate the blood and cause unpleasant symptoms like bloating, water retention, and stubborn-fat gain. If these toxins remain unchecked, they may cause chronic diseases, and even cancer.

7. Control your insulin. Naturally minimize the amount of carbohydrates you ingest by having carbs as the last component of your meal. If needed, supplement yourself with all essential nutrients necessary for stabilizing your insulin, such as essential fatty acids, vitamins, and minerals.

8. Follow a steady exercise routine. A comprehensive diet and exercise routine is the first defense against stubborn fat.

Exercising boosts the metabolic rate, reduces stress-related symptoms, and thus accelerates the diet's effects. However, avoid overtraining. Chronically overstressing your body may cause the opposite effect and slow down your metabolic rate.

Plastic is a very controversial issue. Its use is widespread in packaging all types of food and beverages, and many oils. Most of these plastic bottles are made from polyethylene (a type of plastic that's been shown to be acceptably safe packing material for foods and oils). However, there are plastics used on the market today for packaging food that are toxic.

Udo Erasmus, the "Healthy Fat Guru," says that many plastic fibers contain toxic estrogenic chemicals that are dangerous to our health. In my opinion, avoiding plastic all together would be very impractical and almost impossible today given how widespread it is. Therefore I recommend that everyone do their best to check what type of plastic packaging is used before buying and consuming products wrapped or bottled in them. And, as noted above, you can use your senses. If anything edible smells like plastic, stay away from it. Moreover, acid-based foods, such as lemon juice, vinegar, tomato sauce, and wine shouldn't be packed or stored in plastic containers, since acid is more reactive with certain plastic materials. A few safety measures I use are:

1. Cut away a small amount of the outer edge of foods that are wrapped in plastic, such as cheese.
2. Store food and beverages in glass or ceramic containers.

To sum up how to prevent stubborn fat:

1. Avoid weight fluctuations.
2. Avoid foods you are sensitive or allergic to.
3. Minimize consumption of nonorganic foods.
4. Drink clean, pure water.

5. Avoid foods or liquids that smell like plastic.

6. Avoid excessive alcohol consumption.

7. Control your insulin and minimize carbohydrates.

8. Follow a steady exercise routine.

How to Get Rid of Stubborn Fat

If you suffer from stubborn fat (men usually have it around the belly and the chest; women around their hips, butt, and thighs), and you want to get rid of it, you should also consider trying natural supplements that may help you burn it off.

Natural Stubborn-Fat Busters

Estrogen Blockers: Citrus Bioflavonoids and Soy Flavones

Citrus bioflavonoids contain some natural properties that may block estrogen. Citrus flavonoids are abundant in the white, spongy layer of citrus peels.

Soy flavones contain mild estrogenic properties. It is believed that soy flavones bind to the estrogen receptors in the tissues, and thus block these receptors from estrodiol, the most potent estrogen hormone. Estrodiol is called the "bad estrogen" because of its occasionally powerful effects on the body, such as bloating, water retention, fat gain, feminization of men (such as "bitch tits"), fat under the skin, and stubborn fat gain around the chest and the belly.

Experiments conducted in Italy have shown that combining citrus bioflavonoids with soy flavones was a most powerful, natural way to block the estrogenic effect on the body. Adding citrus bioflavonoids to soy flavones created a more powerful defense against estrogen than taking soy flavones alone.

It's popular today to take soy flavones as a natural preventative aid against estrogen-related cancers, but I feel that a combination of citrus bioflavanoids with stinging nettle and flaxseed lignans is much more potent. Soy flavones may have an estrogenic effect on some people. Let me mention again here that those who are sensitive to soy should consult their physician before taking any supplements containing soy flavones.

Anti–Aromatase Nutrients: Chrysine, Quercetin, Lignans, and Stinging Nettle

Chrysine

Chrysine is a flavone that's derived from the Passiflora plant, or passionflower. It's chemically similar to the flavonoid quercetin.

There was much hype about chrysine a few years ago when it was considered to be a powerful natural anti-aromatase substance. However there are recent studies which question the safety of chrysine. Some researchers believe that it may cause irreversible inhibition of live enzymes.

Quercetin

Quercetin is a flavonoid that serves as a backbone for many other flavonoids including citrus flavonoids. In my opinion, quercetin may work as an anti-aromatase agent if taken in combination with other citrus bioflavanoids. These flavones and flavonoids work very well when combined together. However, when you isolate them they aren't as potent. The synergetic effect of all these flavones together is what makes them so active. That's the way they appear in nature, and that's the best way to take them to get positive results.

Lignans

According to Udo Erasmus, flaxseed lignans, found in the fibrous part of flaxseed, contain anti-estrogenic properties.

It's unclear whether they work by solely blocking estrogen receptors, or by blocking the aromataze enzyme as well. However, lignans have shown positive results as a natural aid against estrogen-related problems. The best way to naturally ingest flaxseed lignans is through high-lignan flaxseed oil, or flaxseed meal. Both are available in health-food stores.

Stinging Nettle

Stinging nettle is an herb with promising potential as a natural aid against aromataze. Historically, people used nettle seeds and roots as a potency herb. Nettle may have an aphrodisiac effect on men by increasing the level of free testosterone in the blood.

The anti-aromatazing properties of this herb are probably due to its ability to bind to the aromataze enzyme, and thus neutralize it. Recent studies suggest the plant may also be useful in treating enlarged prostate. When you take stinging nettle, follow the dosage recommended on the bottle. Nettle may also be a natural aid for women who suffer from estrogen-related stubborn fat. Due to its high-lignan content, this herb may help women block the effect of estrodiol.

Liver Detoxifiers (as Defense Against Alcohol-Related Stubborn Fat and Estrogen Derivatives

Indole-3 Carbinol, Milk Thistle, Dandelion Root, and SAMe

As I've mentioned before, one of the reasons for excessive estrogenic activity in the body is liver congestion. The liver works as a filter organ. It's supposed to break down or neutralize toxins, preventing them from reaching the blood. Excessive alcohol consumption, for instance, blocks the liver enzyme that breaks down estrogen. Therefore, toxic estrogen derivatives go directly into the bloodstream, creating negative estrogenic effects. That's one reason why many heavy drinkers and alcoholics suffer from estrogen-related stubborn fat.

Indole-3 carbinol is a flavon that appears in broccoli, cauliflower, Brussels sprouts, kale, and other cruciferous vegetables. This flavon is believed to be a natural aid for the liver's estrogen metabolism. You would need to ingest a lot of cruciferous vegetables to attain positive results. This may be unappealing, and also uncomfortable, because consuming large amounts of broccoli, for instance, may cause gas, or send you running to the bathroom. It's possible today to buy an active form of inol 3 carbinol, patented as "Dim," and distributed under the brand name Indoplex. Nevertheless, routinely consuming cruciferous vegetables is a natural, simple way to protect the liver. Supplementation is recommended for those who suffer from alcohol-related liver problems. Healthy people, in my opinion, should be able to protect themselves by simply maintaining a proper nutritious diet.

Those who want to accelerate liver detoxification and rejuvenation should consider taking milk thistle and dandelion root, since these herbs have been shown to help the liver detoxify and recuperate. Dandelion root is a diuretic herb and mildly laxative, so be cautious about the amount you take. Start with a small dosage, see how you feel, and then increase it slightly. Both are available as teas, tinctures, and capsules.

Adenosylemethionine (SAMe) is a relatively new supplement. Its primary function is to alleviate depression, however it can also be very useful for liver detoxification, especially for those who suffer from estrogen-related toxicity. Our bodies naturally produce SAMe, but those who have metabolic problems or nutrient deficiencies, may not produce enough. SAMe is available in most health food and specialty vitamin stores.

Those who take steroids, and women who take hormone replacements, place pressure on their liver to break down and detoxify these drugs. An inability by the liver to break them down may cause unpleasant symptoms such as bloating, water retention, and weight gain. Natural supplementation in these cases could help.

Yohimbe bark—Alpha Antagonist

Yohimbe bark is an herb derived from a West African yohimbe tree. Yohimbe is used as an aphrodisiac herb for men who want to boost potency. It may also benefit those who suffer from stubborn fat. Yohimbe is an alpha-2 adrenergenic antagonist, meaning yohimbe may block alpha receptors of fat cells. By blockingalpha-receptors, it makes it possible for a stubborn fat tissue to be metabolized (the adrenal hormones bind to the beta receptors and activate a fat-burning response). For both men and women who suffer from stubborn fat, this herb may offer positive effects. However, some people don't react well to yohimbe. Those who suffer from high-blood pressure, heart conditions, or thyroid problems, should consult their physician before trying it.

To help get rid of stubborn fat, it's worth considering some nutritional supplementation, which may help attack it on four levels:

1. Anti-estrogen (citrus bioflavonoids and flaxseed lignans)
2. Anti-aromatase (quercetin plus citrus bioflavonoids, flaxseed lignans and stinging nettle)
3. Liver detoxifiers (indole-3 carbinol, milk thistle, dandelion root, and SAMe)
4. Alpha antagonist (yohimbe bark)

All the above supplements are available in vitamin and health food stores under different brand names.

Warrior's Stubborn Fat Burner: A Natural Supplement to Block Estrogen-Related Stubborn Fat

A couple of years ago I created a formula that is a potent combination of flavones and herbs that together help rid this fat by blocking the estrogen effect and deactivating alpha receptors on the fat cells. More on this can be found in the "Warrior Nutritional Supplements" chapter

---

The first defense against stubborn fat is to maintain a healthy diet, proper nutrition, and a regular exercise routine. It's best to eat organic foods, drink clean water, try to reduce the purchase, consumption, and storage of foods or liquids packaged in plastic, avoid foods you are sensitive or allergic to, minimize exposure to estrogenic chemicals, minimize your alcohol consumption and, yes, avoid fluctuating your weight through fad or crash diets.

The Warrior Diet can greatly help in preventing and eliminating stubborn fat.

As you've already seen, this diet gives you hours of daily detoxification. This, coupled with the fat burning that happens during the daily Undereating Phase, should keep you lean and healthy. If you are following the overeating rules of the Warrior Diet too, you know that all the nutritional advice mentioned in this chapter is already part of your routine, and so you should be able to block the stubborn-fat syndrome. And, if you have stubborn fat and want to burn it, hopefully you now know what to do.

End Note

As an "End Note" for this subject, let me reiterate how essential exercise is to accelerate fat burning and reduce stress. Of course, maintaining a healthy diet is of utmost importance in order to achieve positive results. Exercise makes the results you're hoping for happen that much faster.

Chapter Eight
The Warrior Diet
Versus Other Diets

I rarely hear people talk about the stability of specific diets, yet, to me, stability is key. Diets have forgotten something I call "Time, the Lost Dimension." We are not steel objects; we are living creatures in time and space. Time is a crucial factor, and can't be ignored. Diets need to reflect the fact that human beings, and all living creatures, exist in time and space, and that we are evolving, moving (or cycling) all the time.

The easiest way to control people is to make them believe they live in a two-dimensional world. But in life, "one plus one" does not always equal "two." Things are built in cycles, due to the time dimension. Life is based on rotations and changes; in the seasons, the weather, day and night. So how can you train people to think that their life should be equal every day?

What I call a stable diet is one that, once you're on it, you can live with on a daily basis. To me, a stable diet isn't just a diet. It's a way of life. So even if you change something, or go off it for a short while, you'll still be balanced. And that's how human beings should be—balanced—whether they eat a little more carbohydrates or protein, or fast, they should still be balanced. That's one motto of the Warrior Diet. Our bodies are built to adapt to various situations without losing homeostasis.

If a diet is built on such specifics that you can easily slip off of it, I call this an "unstable diet." An unstable diet is a bad diet simply because it's almost impossible to stay on it. For instance, The Zone says you should eat 40 percent carbohydrates, 30 percent fat, 30 percent protein, and that if you change the ratio, even slightly, you've lost The Zone. As Barry Sears says, "you're as good as your last meal." To me this diet is the very definition of unstable because, according to its creator, any deviation will mess you up.

Most diets are built on a very simple equation and, to me, this is wrong. These diets can't work for very long because it's impossible to follow a specific, straight formula in an un-straight world. It's just not realistic. You shouldn't eat the same food or ingest the same number of calories every single day because, for instance, some days you do a lot of exercise and others you may not be active at all. You're the same person, but your ratios and needs are changing. Everything in life is evolving. So should your diet.

Light and daylight influence the hormonal system. For some people, there's a peak time of hormone secretion in the afternoon, but for others it's early in the morning. The hormonal system can also be affected if, for instance, you work in the evening as opposed to during the day. Animals and plants are also affected by, and react to, the cycles of day and night and the seasons. Why do we ignore this?

Since the Industrial Revolution, we've been moving further away from the natural cycle of life, governed by sunrise and sunset. As a result, many people today suffer from symptoms of chronic jet lag. Other related problems, like depression or feeling a lack of freedom, are commonplace.

The stability of the Warrior Diet is built on the premise that whether you've eaten your main meal—or if you haven't—you'll always know where you are in the cycle and what you're supposed to do to keep revolving from one part of the cycle to the next.

I believe that nature is very clever, and that we all have deep instincts within us that can provide the wisdom needed about when to eat, when to stop eating, when to fast. Everyone has and needs these cycles, and they differ slightly per individual.

The Warrior Diet allows you to make changes, to binge on carbohydrates or fatty foods like nuts, and still be fine. Other diets don't allow this freedom. I believe that feeling free should be a part of your life. By introducing you to the Warrior Diet, I hope to relay how this sense of freedom will enrich your life in many ways.

The Warrior Diet versus the Frequent-Feeding System

The frequent-feeding system (followed by many people today) is where you eat relatively small, frequent meals throughout the day. Those who advocate frequent feedings say that it puts less pressure on your digestive tract, allegedly keeps sugar levels stable and, especially for body builders and athletes, it enables them to ingest more protein throughout the day to further build muscles.

I understand the philosophy and science behind this, but I also see the down side. With all due respect, the huge disadvantage with the frequent-feeding system is that your body never gets a break to detoxify, to recuperate, and to let the pancreatic system rest. Additionally, when you deposit material so often, without giving your body enough time to detoxify, you basically deplete your body's pool of enzymes. This often results in compromised digestion—especially of proteins. Indigestion weakens the immune system, and if this goes unchecked, leads to diseases.

A large percentage of those who practice the frequent-feeding system no longer have a healthy feeding cycle. It's no wonder so many today suffer from digestive disorders, constipation, and related diseases. These problems are so pronounced that the companies who sell drugs to help people become "regular" make a bloody fortune.

The Warrior Diet is built on daily detoxification with living food enzymes and probiotics as key components. If you practice this diet, you'll eventually reach your own natural cycle and should be able to protect yourself. This makes the Warrior Diet radically different from conventional diets today.

Reviews of Top-Selling Diets, Including How They Differ from the Warrior Diet

I've separated the diet reviews into five major groups:

Group I:
- The All-American Diet
- The American Health-Food Diets

Group II:
- High-Carb/Low-Fat/Low-Protein
- The Pritikin Diet
- Dean Ornish's Diet

Group III:
- The Zone: 40-30-30

Group IV:
- High-Protein, Very Low-Carbohydrate
- Dr. Atkins (New Diet Revolution and Vita-Nutrient Solution)
- Protein Power

Group V:
- Holistic Diets
- Macrobiotics
- Andrew Weil (Instinctive Healing)
- Harvey Diamond (Fit for Life and Fit for Life: A New Beginning)

To make things clear and simple I chose to review only those diets that, in my opinion, best characterize their group.

Group I:

The All-American (Junk Food) Diet— from hot dogs and french fries to sodas, chips and cookies.

There are no books in this category, other than cookbooks (and fast-food or diner menus).

This is a relatively young diet, less than a hundred years old. It cropped up during the twentieth century, and is an example of what I call a "scavenger diet." People on this diet don't think about what they eat, and blithely consume prepared and overly processed foods. True scavengers don't hunt for food; they eat what's left over by another animal. They pick up and eat dead food. Scavengers have their own mentality.

The All-American Diet is based on consuming food without considering its nutritional value. This is a very aggressive diet, high in refined and overly processed foods loaded with preservatives, nitrates, and artificial food colors. When I say aggressive, I refer to taste—meaning there's too much sugar, too much salt, and grease. Sugar overstimulates your insulin levels, and keeps you craving more of it. Overly processed foods, like hot dogs, cold cuts, cakes, cookies, candies, sodas, and other sugar-laden beverages, refined or sugary grains like most muffins, donuts, and cereals, French fries (and all fried foods), make up the majority of the All-American Diet.

Many of you already know how bad this diet is. Much data show its correlation to diabetes, heart attacks, and degenerative diseases. It's my contention that even if you try to balance it somewhat by reducing your sugar consumption and increasing your use of olive oil, instead of margarine or other hydrogenated oils, you're still left with too much overly processed food. To add insult to injury, unless you eat organically, much of the food is contaminated with petroleum-based chemicals, hormones, antibiotics, and estrogenic derivatives. You can't win here!

The American "Health Food" Diets

Choosing organic food is definitely a step in the right direction, because it means you're paying some attention to what you eat. You're attempting to avoid the hormones and antibiotics found in most nonorganic meats and dairy products, as well as the chemically-laden herbicides, pesticides, and fertilizers used in most of the nation's food supply.

But one of the common mistakes people make when they see a health-food label, is going for it without checking the ingredients. A lot of organic foods, including many cereals, contain too much sugar or other sweeteners, like fructose, or have undesirable oils or overly processed fats--all of which, research has shown as unhealthy and therefore dangerous to your health.

Group II:

High-Carbohydrate, Low-Fat, Low-Protein.

The Pritikin Diet and Dean Ornish's diet belong here. This group is still the most popular today, despite massive research showing the insulin impact of carbohydrate-based diets.

High-carb, low-fat, low-protein diets have proven ineffective in terms of weight loss. Even when calories are reduced, many who try these diets gain weight. Following high-carb, low-fat, low-protein diets can also lead to major problems. For example, when there's a chronic imbalance between protein and carbohydrate consumption, where you eat an excessive amount of carbs and don't ingest adequate amounts of protein, it may result in protein deficiencies, as well as place too much pressure on your pancreas to produce insulin. This can, in turn, lead to insulin insensitivity, hypoglycemia, and even diabetes. Additionally, active people require more protein than those who are sedentary. These diets may not supply enough amino acids for their active muscles.

It's common to find people with "Fat Phobias" in this territory. When you don't consume enough healthy fats, especially essential fatty acids (EFA's), you may suffer from an EFA deficiency. An EFA deficiency may lead to metabolic problems in the brain, body tissues, in the cellular level, and compromise all bodily systems.

Moreover, it may lead to depression, impotency, and eventually full-blown diseases.

Group III:

The Zone (40/30/30)

I respect many of Barry Sears' theories, and he's made a great step ahead by explaining to people the mechanism of fat burning and the difference between insulin and glucagon. However, there's absolutely no reason to conclude from his theory that there is actually a "Zone."

In my opinion, if there is something similar to the alleged Zone, it definitely doesn't look like the Zone. I can prove philosophically, not just scientifically, how wrong this assumption is. First of all, let's address the amount and proportion of food. There's no proof that all people should consume 40 percent carbs, 30 percent protein, and 30 percent fat daily.

He's made two wrong assumptions. One, he believes that this ratio fits everybody—men and women of different ages, athletes, and sedentary people. The truth is that different people have different needs, so you can't say that everybody should follow the same ratio. Moreover, some people suffer from metabolic problems such as gout or hypoglycemia, and their diet absolutely must accommodate their condition. Secondly, Sears ignores the fact that a diet's protein-to-carb ratio depends on your goal. If you're in a phase where you want to lose weight, you should have one ratio; if you want to maintain your weight, you should have another.

To me, the worst thing about the Zone is that it's built, like all diets I'm aware of today, on control and deprivation. The human instinct to reach satiety (satisfaction) from food, and to have a sense of freedom, cannot be achieved with this diet. Maybe people can fool themselves for a while, but the fact that you have to measure everything, almost like a pharmacist, is very difficult for people to maintain. I think the Zone is a potentially interesting diet, and some people can probably lose weight on it. But for those who want to build lean tissues, whileboosting their metabolism and feeling a sense of freedom and satisfaction from their meals, I believe the Zone diet is just not good enough.

Group IV:

High-Protein, Low- or No-Carbohydrates diets, including Dr. Atkins' New Diet Revolution and Vita-Nutrient Solution, Protein Power, and The Carbohydrate Addict's Diet.

I chose to review Dr. Atkins' New Diet Revolution and Vita-Nutrient Solution for Group IV because I feel it represents this group well.

Dr. Atkins is a pioneer, since he was the first to seriously introduce to the public the science behind fat burning, as well as the hazards of carbohydrates and overconsumption of sugar. But, unfortunately, his diet suffers from the same problem as The Zone. I believe it's impossible to follow his diet for the long term because you can't ask people to deprive themselves of carbs forever. There are other problems too, involving overacidity and imbalance, by not consuming enough raw plant foods, and over-consumption of protein and fatty foods, such as hot dogs, cold cuts, or bacon, which acidify the body and deplete it from its vital enzymes. On top of this, Dr. Atkins disregards the importance of whole foods and their healing effects on the body. The emphasis on live, raw foods is missing from his diet plan. Human beings were created as an integral part of nature, and consuming whole foods is essential for our health.

In his latest book, Dr. Atkins' Vita-Nutrient Solution, he suggests a list of vitamins and herbs that you can take to supplement this high protein, high-fat, low-carbohydrate diet. I feel he has drawn the wrong conclusions. Chronically avoiding carbs may compromise the body's natural production of serotonin, a major neurotransmitter that triggers pleasure sensors in the brain, giving a calming effect as well as feelings of satisfaction and happiness. My contentions are that:

- There is no substitute for the phytonutrients, minerals, and vitamins we get from whole foods.
- Whole carbs should be an essential component of the diet.

Recommending to cut out some of which nature provides—fruits, plants, whole grains and fibers—and instead use synthetic supplements is absolutely wrong. Phytonutrients, minerals, and microorganisms are needed to support your bodily functions and hormones, even potentiate vitamins and support your glands. The Atkins Diet misses a lot of potent, living-food forces.

The colors of live food, such as the pigments in plants, are actually nutritious and essential for your health. Some are flavones or other organic compounds, which support the human system. These phytonutrients are much more potent in their natural state than in synthetic forms. You can't just supplement them with processed powders.

Many years ago, when the soil was richer and less contaminated with environmental toxins, food contained quite a few more flavones and phytonutrients, which supported our bodies hormonal and metabolic systems. Their decline in our food supply is an overall problem today. So why follow a diet that makes this problem more pronounced?

Dr. Atkins almost completely ignores the importance of natural detoxification, the role of living food and food enzymes. I believe, moreover, that following this high-protein, high-fat diet with the absence of daily detoxification will place too much pressure on the liver, and so will eventually toxify your body, and increase the effects of aging. Atkins' slogan that "you can eat whatever protein and fat that you want," including bacon, salami, cheese, and butter, is a dangerous gimmick. If you choose to go on this gimmicky diet, you may temporarily lose weight, but eventually will have the health of a sausage.

In summary, the Atkins' diet lacks three major things:

- The importance of the wholeness of food, derived primarily from plants and some grains.
- Daily detoxification
- A sense of freedom, since it's built on deprivation.

Group V: HOLISTIC DIETS

- **Macrobiotic Diets**
- **Andrew Weil's Instinctive Healing**
- **Harvey Diamond's Fit For Life and Fit For Life: A New Beginning.**

Macrobiotics

Macrobiotic diets are based on the ancient Chinese concept of balancing yin and yang. However, this is an American modern mutation of an old Chinese tradition. These diets are based mainly on consumption of cooked food, including cooked fruits and veggies. Grains are the main source of energy.

Yin foods are those that have light, expansive, and often cooling properties, such as fruits, vegetables, sugar, and some herbs and spices. Yang foods have contractive, anabolic, and often warming qualities, such as meat, grains, and beans. Since macrobiotic diets are vegetarian, the yang foods are mainly grains, nuts, seeds, beans and legumes.

In my opinion, these diets aren't as balanced as they claim to be. They neglect, or nearly avoid, the living-food factor. As a result, people who eat a macrobiotic diet miss the live-food factors, which as mentioned, are so essential for your health. I also argue the wisdom of balancing the yin and yang food with each meal. Some people are more acidic, so they need more yin, alkalizing food, and the opposite holds true, too. Moreover, cooking methods may change the quality of fresh yin-like food into a more yang-like quality. It's confusing. On top of all this, it's simply impractical to follow, especially for people who are on the run. Macrobiotic junkies usually carry pre-cooked food with them in plastic containers. This is inconvenient; furthermore, precooked food may spoil if left for too long without refrigeration. This diet is built on control and deprivation because your choices are limited, and you can't use your own instincts freely. As I've said before: no freedom, no good!

Andrew Weil's Instinctive Healing

I respect Andrew Weil. He is a brilliant man and deserves the credit for educating people about the importance of fresh food, the dangers of processing, and making the right choices when it comes to different plants, seeds, and herbs. Dr. Weil puts things in the right perspective when he covers the subjects of healthy oils and natural toxins. He also elaborates wisely about different healthy cooking methods, and the importance of being in tune with nature and seasons when it comes to your diet.

But philosophy is one thing, and a practical diet is another. I suspect that one of Dr. Weil's magic bullets, besides his charisma, is his ability to remove guilt from those who are looking for guidance. Using Weil himself as a living example of his diet philosophy is somewhat confusing. Dr. Weil argues that the lean body image isn't a healthy one. According to him it's all right to be chunky (like himself), and this point of view suggests to people that it's okay to be a roly-poly. Dr. Weil says bodybuilding is bad for you, and that moving yourself from the chair to the kitchen and back is kind of an exercise (well, maybe gardening and walking is mentioned, too). I find this approach to be misleading. People can do better than that. In short, if you want to follow Andrew Weil, you may learn a lot about food and cooking. But you might find yourself looking like, well, Andrew Weil.

Harvey Diamond's Fit for Life and Fit for Life: A New Beginning

These diets are very popular among those people who are looking for a practical way to heal themselves.

Harvey Diamond's books are built on three major premises:

1. Food Separation—Carbohydrate and protein meals should be separated. According to Diamond, food separation will guarantee better digestion since carbs and protein need different enzymes under different pH.

2. Detoxification—In his latest book, Fit For Life: A New Beginning, Diamond elaborates on the importance of periodic lymphatic system detoxification as the only natural way to prevent disease.

3. Living Food—Diamond explains the vital importance of living food forces as an integral part of the diet.

My main problem with these books was, and I say was, that in my opinion they appeal to sick or sedentary people. I fully understand and agree with his suggestion of consuming fruits and freshly squeezed fruit and veggie juices, but disagree with the part concerning what and how much you're allowed to eat. I, as well as other active people, would literally disappear if I followed Fit for Life. However, after speaking with and meeting Harvey Diamond, I realize that he's much more flexible than I thought before we met. Harvey agreed that his diet doesn't target active people or athletes who need to consume more protein and meat. He admits that in spite of his attack on "flesh foods," he no longer is a vegetarian, and does, in fact, enjoy a steak once in a while.

Given the above, I have to say that this is a diet I honestly recommend as one of the most effective means of detoxification, for healing and breaking old, unhealthy habits. I personally don't follow food separation since I feel that eating carbs alone may cause a rapid rise in insulin, while combining protein, fat, and carbs in one meal prevents high-insulin fluctuations—and has the added benefit of providing more satiety. Further, some natural whole foods, such as beans and nuts, contain both protein and carbohydrates in almost the same ratio.

Let me just note that Harvey is also a great writer with a wonderful sense of humor. He cracked me up a few times. No other diet book has ever made me laugh.

Chapter Nine
Lessons from History

The mighty Roman soldier was a lightweight (135 lbs.) on average). Yet in face-to-face combat against Gauls or Celts who weighed about 180 lbs., the Roman warrior came out on top. Julius Caesar was only 5 ft. 6 in. tall, and Alexander the Great wasn't physically a big man, but history remembers them as giant warriors.

One might ask why history remembers these lean people as giants. In my opinion, the answer lies somewhere between the ways these people lived, and how adamantly they followed their convictions.

I've chosen to focus mainly on the ancient Romans and Greeks for two reasons. First, the Greco-Roman culture is considered the foundation of modern Western civilization. Western cultural ideals of beauty and body proportions are derived from the Greco-Roman classical period.

Secondly, I find the Greeks, and especially the Romans, great historical examples of people who created large empires and documented their warrior way of life over hundreds of years.

There's a lot to learn from ancient warriors, but since this isn't a history book, I have limited myself to major topics relevant to the Warrior Diet. To understand what made these people live as they did, you need to get acquainted with their priorities. What were their aesthetic and moral concepts of beauty and ugliness? What did courage and cowardice mean to them? How did they relate to subjects such as health and sickness? And, especially, what were their attitudes toward pain, pleasure, deprivation, and compensation? I find it all most intriguing. Hopefully, you will too.

Although I focus mainly on the Romans and Greeks, I do refer to other groups of ancient people as well. I hope this perspective will shed some light on the historical relevance of the Warrior Diet.

At the end of the chapter I offer my conclusions and elaborate on the historical role of nutritional carbohydrates.

An Empire of Wanderers

Romans devoured space. They spent most of their lives outdoors. They traveled the length and breadth of Latium, Italy, and the provinces (the regions that were conquered by the Romans, such as Gaul, North Africa, and Palestine) as soldiers, magistrates, or freed men entrusted with their patron's business.

"On the move," they had to be constantly alert and able to adapt to different foods, weather conditions, and especially to times of deprivation. It was essential for nomadic people to maintain a practical diet, which could keep them moving from one place to another. They were, therefore, geared towards accessible seasonal fresh food, as well as using natural preservation methods for their food supply. As you'll soon see, diet and food supply played quite a large role in their lives. Maintaining a healthy food supply required special strategies. These strategies influenced almost every aspect of their lives, including how they planned war campaigns.

What You See Is What You Get

Physical appearance was crucial to all Romans. They conducted business face-to-face. Army commanders had to stand before their soldiers and demonstrate physical and rhetorical authority. A positive self-image was an essential factor that could never be taken for granted.

Roman awareness of self was derived from the way others looked at them. Their virtues and vices were an open book, and were manifest in their style of dress, tone of voice, and choice of body movements. They were forever on stage, but always played themselves. Judged by their physical appearance, those who neglected it were no longer respected as citizens or men. To look at a man was to know the truth about him.

The famous censor, Cato, wore a close-fitting toga. When giving speeches, he did so with deliberate delivery, few gestures, and careful steps. Thus he would exemplify his political program: *austerity and restraint.*

Roman people had a very strict, aesthetic concept of physical appearance. They had their own unique style, which they called cultus. Cultus involved body washing, hairstyling, beard trimming and, especially, eating adequately. To suspend one's body cultus demonstrated *self-neglect.* Gluttony was considered a disgrace, and obesity a humiliating weakness. Censors debarred obese cavalrymen from the army. In order to look lean, Romans had to maintain a special diet. This diet had unique rules, which I'll cover later on.

Attention paid to physical appearance was evident among Spartan warriors, too. According to Plutarch, Spartans kept their hair long, as they believed that long hair made a strong man look handsome. A shaved head was a sign of defeat and failure. A "skinhead" was a loser. Greeks idealized physical appearance and class. This is apparent when one looks at the way their artists portrayed Olympian athletes, heroes, and gods in paintings and sculpture.

The ancient Greeks had a common saying: "Tell me what you eat, with whom and how, and I will tell you who you are!"

A Soldier's Status

Roman soldiers had to take an oath (*Sacramentum*). This Sacramentum released them from the prohibitions and constraints of civilian life. They wore clothing different from civilian men; soldiers didn't wear togas or light colored garments. They wore dark red tunics that wouldn't show bloodstains.

Being a soldier required a total commitment to obey orders, and kill or die for a cause. The hardship of military life, battle wounds, and the scars of war were all a source of pride. Soldiers enjoyed a high status, and were respected accordingly.

Great philosophers, historians, and orators were involved one way or another with soldiers and warriors. Aristotle (384–322

B.C.) was a tutor of Alexander the Great. Xenophon (428–354 B.C.), a leading associate of Socrates, was an Athenian mercenary in the Persian army under Cyrus the Younger. Demosthenes (384–322 B.C.), the last spokesman of free Athens, was a lifelong opponent of Philip of Macedonia and his son, Alexander the Great. He committed suicide with poison. Philosophy and spirituality went hand in hand with the sword. Warriors surrounded themselves with philosophers and tutors, and spiritual leaders were ready to sacrifice their lives for their ideas.

Sense of Chivalry

One element of the Warrior Instinct, manifested throughout history, was the way men carried arms to defend themselves, their honor, as well as the honor of their loved ones. Males were routinely trained from a young age to acquire fighting skills, such as fencing, wrestling, and later, shooting. During the Greco-Roman period, it was the right and privilege of free people to carry arms. Dueling was popular among free men since biblical times. American statesman Alexander Hamilton, and the Russian poet Pushkin, both died in duels while defending their honor. Dueling was an accepted part of life until the twentieth century.

Virtues and Vices

Courage, generosity, devotion, and self-sacrifice were traits adored in the Greco-Roman society. Cowardice, according to the Romans, was to be treated with cruelty. The Romans were driven to be adventurous, take risks, and were tempted to gamble just to see how far they could venture without tipping over. Being adventurous was regarded as a courageous way of life. Adventure stories of warriors who wandered to remote and dangerous places were part of Roman and Greek mythology. The Warrior Instinct, which drives people to take risks and even put themselves in life danger, was an immanent part of life.

Self-control was a matter of life and death in the ancient Roman world. Sensual passions and overindulgence were considered serious weaknesses, which threatened to dissolve the body. Ancient Greeks and Romans believed heroism protected them from death. Let me point out here that the ability to withstand pain, hunger, and fear were thought to be the warrior's main strength. For the Romans, war was a "competition of pain." Those who could withstand the most suffering would win.

Since pain and deprivation were an integral part of warrior life, they would induce both in order to conquer fears and be tough enough to withstand the hardship of war. Army leaders, such as Pompey and Mucius Scaevola, also physically tortured themselves.

The Greco-Roman Warrior Cycle

Romans cycled between extremities of deprivation and compensation. A typical cycle was based on intense activity during the day, and relaxation during the night. There was also a yearly cycle, based on the seasons:

• Spring through summer was the time for war and work.

• Winter was the time for peace.

• Autumn was the time of transition between war and peace. This was the season for "the Games."

Each cycle had its rules. Following them was not an option. It was a must.

Romans and Greeks were very conscious of different classes in society, and each class, whether rich, poor, freed men, or slaves had their own rules. To keep things simple, I'll cover the most dominant rules and social behaviors.

As you'll see, poor people had a different diet from the elite. You'll also note that hard laborers and soldiers, who were engaged in extreme physical activities, needed to satisfy their high-calorie demands by consuming carbohydrates during the day. However, during peacetime, consumption of carbs was minimized to raw foods such as veggies or fruits.

Food prohibitions were enacted to enforce diet rules, especially during wartime. This meant that certain luxury foods were not allowed for sale on days other than festivals. Caesar sent special supervising brigades to the markets to seize foods in violation of the law. Soldiers broke into houses to check what was being served in people's dining rooms. During wartime, there was a maximum annual sum that citizens could spend on luxuries such as bacon or salty meat.

Daytime Activities

Daytime was dedicated to work and war. A Roman had to struggle throughout the day, dealing with physical stress and anxiety. Being alert was part of the daily routine. Luxuries, pleasures, and ostentation were not allowed.

The only function of food during the day was to restore strength. People ate standing up. In times of necessity, such as during war campaigns, soldiers ate only dry biscuits and water. Given this, Romans in general didn't like dry food; they ate it for nourishment only. When people traveled, they often ate bread and figs, as they didn't have the time or facilities to cook meals.

Poor people, and those unwilling to wait until the evening meal, would gnaw at dry bread, boiled vegetable leftovers, or an onion. The poor were often on the brink of starvation; eating during the day was for them a matter of survival. The elite ate only one meal, at night. They minimized food consumption during the day to mainly crudus (raw, uncooked foods).

Evening Pleasures

The evening was dedicated to relaxation, pleasure, and socialization, including family gatherings. This time was organized around the evening meal, called the "Cena."

Roman citizens went to public baths in the early evening. Taking a bath was a transition ritual between the physical agitation and anxiety of the day, and the evening leisure, or "Otium."

It was essential for people to relax at night and avoid all signs of being troubled or worried. They did not talk business. The wealthy had their slaves play music. Those who couldn't relax were thought to be suffering from a stiff or corrupted soul. Given all these relaxation rules, Romans, with their warrior discipline, always retained a certain alertness. They sat on Roman chairs, which had no back, and forced them to remain alert.

The evening relaxation prepared them for sleep. Sleep was essential for a Roman who had to awaken at dawn. Insomnia was considered a sign of weakness, remorse, regret, worry, longing or having a bad conscience.

Concept of Food

The Roman concept of food was both symbolic and sensual. According to their beliefs, *crudus* (raw food) was considered animal fodder. They felt that if a man ate the same raw food which wild animals ate, he might himself turn into a beast. In spite of the fact that Romans felt this way, they ate crudus during the day as part of the daytime austerity.

Romans believed strongly in "Humanitas" – human feeling and culture. Food, therefore, was prepared in ways that would differentiate it from its raw state. Romans preferred soft foods. To them soft foods were the opposite of crude, tough to chew, raw, and therefore "animalistic" foods. During the Cena, food was cooked, eaten warm, and, of better quality.

The Plebeian Diet

The plebeian diet was based mainly on grains and legumes. Meat, cheese, fish, seafood, and eggs were available, but only rich people could afford them on a regular basis. I must mention here that poor and working-class Romans liked to eat cheese, seafood, and bacon if accessible and affordable, but were generally forced to compromise, and so consumed a principally vegetarian diet of mainly grains. As a result they often suffered from protein deficiencies. To get enough protein, they combined grains with legumes; beans and peas were their main sources of protein. They prepared grains and beans using two methods:

Grinding it into flour and baking it; and cooking it in water.

Basic Food Preparations

A cooked meal—"Gruel"—consisted of grains mixed with legumes, pieces of meat or fish, all boiled together in water for a long time. Romans preferred boiling to roasting or grilling because boiling adds water to the food, and softens it.

Oil was used and consumed only during the evening meal. Fresh olive oil was added to bean purees, gruel, meat, and dry cheese.

I find it interesting to note that army rations of wine and beer in early modern Europe were pretty high. For instance, daily rations of wine for the Spanish navy during the sixteenth century were 1.14 liters per soldier. Daily rations of beer and wine for Russian army soldiers in the eighteenth century were 3.5 liters and 0.25 liters, respectively. A British seaman during the Napoleonic wars enjoyed a daily ration of up to 4.5 liters of beer. Looking at these rations may make one wonder about the role alcohol played in historical war campaigns.

Soldiers also liked to fortify their carb meals with protein. Mixing protein, fat, and carbohydrates all together was generally preferred to eating carbs alone.

Wining and Dining in Ancient Rome

Dining

Free Romans did not dine with slaves. Slaves and hard laborers ate during the day. Cato fed his slaves barley, fermented fish, olives, and vinegar. During seasons of particularly hard labor, workers ate bread shaped like a dough ball, with cheese and honey in the center.

Romans liked to eat with company. Eating alone was considered unwelcome and depressing.

Wining

Romans liked to drink wine. Wine was diluted with (sometimes warm and salty) water to reduce its acidity: one part wine to two parts of water, or the opposite.

The greatest warriors in history, Alexander the Great and Julius Caesar, drank a lot of wine. Most warriors, in fact, drank wine, and the more they wandered, the more they drank. Roman warriors liked wine and beer.

According to the Greek historian Thucydides (c.460–400 B.C.), Spartan soldiers enjoyed a steady supply of both wine and meat. Great mythological heroes like Hercules, and the God of Wine, Dionysus, were notorious for their gargantuan drinking habits. Even the Bible regards wine as a source of happiness.

The Meal "Cena"

The Cena evening meal was designed to include three courses. The first course was *'Gustatio'* (taster or appetizer). Gustatio was meant to introduce a variety of tastes and textures. A typical appetizer was a combination of honeyed wine, mixed with tasty small tidbits. Roman cooks mixed ground seafood with exotic herbs and oil to create an unrecognizable, mysterious, and tasty appetizer. Gustatio was made in different varieties, such as boiled eggs and olives (egg salad), or bacon, walnuts, and dried figs taken from the cellar.

The second, or main, course typically included wild boar, turbot fish, plump chicken—all very well cooked, until the meat fell apart. There was a kind of food hierarchy in regard to evening meals:

- The bottom level consisted of grains, legumes, vegetables, fruits, oil, and wine
- The middle level was based on cooked farm-raised animals
- The top (preferred) level was a meal that included wild game, boar, or hare

The most popular fish sauce was *garum*—fermented fish mixed with salt and herbs.

Since Romans liked soft food, the most popular evening meals were prepared by mixing vegetables with different ingredients such as grains, lentils, meat, fish or cheese into one mushy, soft, warm serving. This whole meal included a variety of tastes and textures to satisfy and relax the diner.

Extreme luxury foods for Romans included fatty meats, fish, eel, and especially shellfish. Roman nobles had their own fishponds (*piscinae*) where they cultivated fish and shellfish for their own use.

The third course was dessert. Desserts were chiefly based on fresh fruits such as apples, grapes, or figs. Sometimes they consumed their favorite delicacies, such as shrimp, oysters, or snails, as a condiment to finish the meal.

Mixing Carbs and Protein

Those following the Warrior Diet who choose to mix carbs with protein for the main meal can do so as long as the carbs *are not eaten before* the protein. However, those interested in losing body fat should consume carbs as the last component of the meal. In so doing, the quantity of carbs consumed will be minimized naturally without restriction. This method also helps regulate the amount of carbs ingested when cycling between days of high protein meals and days of high carb meals.

Carb Content in Ancient Warrior Meals

The ideal ancient warrior meal consisted mainly of animal proteins, such as meat, fish, eggs, and cheese. Carbs were a secondary component, meant to add texture and bulk to the cooked food. However, in reality, soldiers were often forced to use carbs as a main source of food because of shortages in animal proteins. Soldiers generally needed more carbs than civilians to satisfy their high calorie and energy expenditures.

Rules of Eating

There were a few rules—or customs—that had to be followed during the meal.

1. Introduce all tastes

Appetizers (*gustatio*) were served at the beginning of the meal to introduce a variety of tastes before the main course. The appetizers were very small, and their function was for taste and pleasure only. Roman cooks used leeks, sorrel, salt, pepper, and cumin for gustatio.

"High-Sky Foods"

Romans believed that natural energy existed within some raw foods. They believed, for instance, that berries contained sun energy, and therefore these fruits were considered to be "high sky." Sun-strong foods had to be eaten on an empty stomach in order to keep the right energy flow. Too much energy, according to the Romans, was not thought to be good, as they felt it would put one out of balance.

Berries and sun-dried fruits were therefore generally consumed on an empty stomach. For example, mulberries picked before the sun was too high in the sky were to be eaten on an empty stomach during the day.

2. Start with subtle-tasting foods, and move to more aggressive tastes

Salads were introduced in the beginning of the meal, and not brought out with the wine, which was mainly drunk toward the end of the meal. Falandrian wine (wine that came from Falandria, a Roman region, that was notorious for its strong taste) was not served at the beginning of the meal because it was too strong to drink on an empty stomach. Roman condiments, mostly spicy, with a strong or sweet taste, were served at the end.

3. After the meal—relaxation

Relaxation after the meal was a must. People would converse. Philosophical, spiritual, and intellectual ideas were discussed. The atmosphere and mood was care- and worry-free. Roman people liked humor, especially at night. Music, dancing, and poetry were popular as well.

Elimination

Healthy digestion and elimination were a necessity of warrior life. Being regular was, therefore, already a priority a couple of thousand years ago. Romans used different preparations of mussels, other shellfish, and sorrel cooked in wine from Chios, to make an effective laxative.

Since the plebeian diet was rich in natural fiber—whether cooked or raw—it is reasonable to conclude that they didn't use laxatives. Moreover, they couldn't afford them. I assume that the popularity of these laxative food preparations among the elite Romans was because their main meal was high in protein and relatively low in fiber.

On another note, Alexander the Great is believed to be the first Westerner to have discovered the banana, in India. He originally thought the banana was a type of fig. After his soldiers ate some overripe bananas and suffered from diarrhea, Alexander issued an executive order to avoid them. For the Macedonians, bananas were forbidden because warriors were not supposed to put themselves at risk to suffer from bloating or any other unpleasant digestive symptoms that could slow them down.

Balancing Overindulgence

Romans treated overindulgence, and its presumed consequence, weight gain, in a variety of ways, such as exercising outdoors, collecting wood, digging, running into the Campus Martius, or taking a dip in the freezing Tiber river. These people had an almost obsessive way of creating checks and balances to their physical and mental states.

Sickness and Medicine

Sick people were suspected of having committed a morally weak action. Romans were extremely superstitious. As advanced as they were in science, politics, and art, they strongly believed in signs,

signs, luck, curses, and blessings. Both Romans and Greeks were pagans. Every Roman home had a god or goddess to protect their family. They also strongly believed in "what you see is what you get." In their eyes, morality and physical health went hand-in-hand.

Traditional Roman healing remedies included:

- Fasting—to heal stomach troubles

- Pomegranate extract—for colic and worms

- Cabbage—According to Cato, cabbage was a universal remedy for almost every illness. Treats such as fried cabbage were used to heal insomnia. The popular "cabbage soup diet" is as old as the Roman Empire.

- Music—For the Romans, music was a most powerful healing aid. The Greeks believed that music could bring the muse of gods to humans. According to Socrates, music was the ultimate art, which brought forth the ideas of harmony, beauty, and health.

Roman Health

Romans were generally in good shape. A Roman soldier, who spent most of his adult life in the army, was able to physically endure for long periods of time, especially during army campaigns. An infantryman had to carry 40–60 lbs. of equipment on his back, march thirty miles, toil, build camps or fight—almost every day. To withstand such physical and mental demands, a Roman warrior obviously had to be in a good state of health.

The majority of health problems that civilian Romans suffered from at that time were related to protein, vitamin, and mineral deficiencies. Ailments such as eye infections, stomach aches, skin disorders, summer and autumn fever, were mostly related to nutrient deficiencies. The high-grain, low-protein vegetarian diet of the poor often caused protein deficiencies, particularly so for children and pregnant women.

Plebeian Roman diets, high in wheat, and lower-strata Greek, particularly Spartan, diets that were high in barley were deficient in the protein lysine, vitamins A, C, and D and in certain minerals such as zinc. The shortage of animal food and consumption of high-phytate grains (bread or cereal) caused mineral deficiencies, such as iron and calcium. I can list more vitamin and mineral deficiencies, and the symptoms of the above deficiencies. But, since this isn't a history or medical book, I've just outlined some general problems of the time, and how people tried to deal with them.

Diet and Nutrition

Beans: The Main Source of Protein

As mentioned, the typical plebeian diet was based on grains. To avoid protein deficiencies, they mixed grains with legumes. Beans were considered "the poor man's meat." They were also the gladiator's main source of protein, as well as Roman soldiers in times of short supply of meat, cheese, or fish. The bean was a strong symbol. It conjured up images of death, hell, blood, and semen, but yet at the same time was considered a good-luck charm.

There were rules for consuming beans. Romans were aware that they caused gas, bloating, and water retention. In time they developed techniques for cooking beans to reduce, or eliminate, these side effects. Techniques included triple rinsing, then soaking in water overnight, than triple rinsing again, and finally peeling and removing their skin—all before cooking.

Poor people ate beans as part of the main meal. Roman soldiers mixed bean flour with wheat or barley to enrich bread. The wealthy ate beans and other plebeian food to affirm their superiority over the lower classes. They used beans as a condiment. The "elite bean treat" was served at the end of the meal and resembled baked beans mixed with honey. For the Greeks, beans were a symbol of democracy. However, the Greeks preferred oligarchy. They considered democracy the rule of the partly because of oligarchy. Like the wealthy Romans, wealthy Greeks ate beans as special dishes only. They ate young, fresh beans, which were soft and tender, as desserts (*tragema*) or in the form of soup or exotic sauces.

Grains

Wheat was the Roman soldiers' main source of grain. For the Greeks and Spartans, it was barley. Roman warriors' rations were about 800g–1000g of grain daily. During campaigns, a soldier's diet was made up of 80 percent grain and 20 percent other foods such as meats, cheese, legumes, and veggies. According to this it appears that an average Roman soldier consumed about 3,000 calories of grains alone per day.

In my opinion, these calorie figures could be misleading. The soldiers used to carry hand mills with them to grind their own flour on a daily basis. Part of this flour was used to bake dry biscuits to be used during the day. Reluctant as the Romans normally were to consume dry food, these biscuits were more for back up and would frequently have been discarded. The Roman warrior preference was for high protein foods.

Wheat and barley are, of course, relatively high in protein and were, therefore, superior to other grains and carbohydrates such as polished rice (which was consumed by many Asians) and roots (consumed by many Africans). Rice and roots are short not only in protein, but other vital nutrients, too. Those who lived on such sources of carbohydrates alone suffered from severe protein deficiencies.

Other Foods (Protein and Oil)

The basic diet of both Roman and Greek commoners was vegetarian (but not exclusively). When these people had access to meat, fish, or cheese they preferred it.

- Meat: The most popular meat for Greeks was goat. For Romans, it was pork.

- Dairy and milk: Came mostly from sheep and goats. Romans did not use butter.
- Olive oil: Was freshly squeezed, to avoid rancidity. It was used as an alternative to butter and soap.
- Fish: Was domestic, and both fresh and saltwater fish were consumed.
- Poultry: Was eaten occasionally, whenever available.

Commoners' Diet

Pliny the Elder wrote that Romans consumed more meat than the Athenians, particularly pork. Poor people could only occasionally afford to purchase meat, sausages, or blood puddings of dubious content in the sundry cook shops in the city. Choicer food was sometimes available at public festivals. But such events were not frequent enough to have made much difference nutritionally.

Common people would eat chickpeas (like today's popcorn) in theaters. Hot "peace pudding" made of chickpeas was sold cheaply on the streets. Poor people could occasionally afford cheap vegetables such as cabbage, leeks, beets, garlic, and onions. They might, at times, have also consumed cheap fish from polluted sections of the Tiber, old smelly fish, small-fry, and low-quality fish sauce. To compensate for a shortage in animal protein consumption, the poor ate legumes, which supplied vitamin A, as well as the amino acids that are low in wheat and barley.

Soldiers' Meals

The quickest and easiest way to prepare a soldier's meal was to cook porridge (a mixture of grains, veggies, legumes, and, if accessible, meat or fish boiled in water). It did not require much time to build a fire or to make the porridge. Soldiers occasionally fortified bread by adding bean flour to the grains. Herodian reported that warriors typically made barley cakes and baked them on charcoal. Biscuits were specially prepared breads that were very dry, and could be kept for long periods

Soldiers prepared their own meals. Basic units were called the "*Contubernium.*" They were made up of between eight to ten soldiers, who shared a tent, and took care of their own daily needs. Soldiers ate at night after toiling and building camps. Nighttime was the best time for cooking and especially baking, which required camping facilities and time. During army campaigns, soldiers had to prepare quick meals. Each meal had to satisfy the warriors nutritional and caloric needs.

Living off the Land

Macedonian, Spartan, and Roman warriors lived off the land. Foraging was a fundamental part of warfare, and armies had to rely on local food supplies. A Roman legion of 5,000 soldiers needed to feed almost 10,000 people, including servants, slaves, and allied soldiers. The daily burden of an average Roman army added up to shiploads of wheat and barley, herds of cattle, and wagonloads of wine, vinegar, and olive oil. Transportation of large amounts of food made it difficult for an army on the move to conduct an efficient war campaign, especially on the mainland. A dependence on transporting the food supply slowed the advance of an army, and sometimes brought it to a halt.

Tactical strength was a necessity to successfully live off the land. Warriors had to be aware of the seasons when different crops would be available. Choosing the right season could play a major role in whether a military campaign was successful. Greek historian Polybius describes the successful gathering of wheat by Hannibal (during July–August) near Gerunium during the Carthaginian campaign against the Romans.

Training to live off the land began at a young age for Spartan boys. They were taught to look for food outdoors during the seasons they could find it, and these hungry boys would steal food if necessary in order to survive. If caught, they were punished. This preparation also triggered their Warrior Instinct, as they became adept at cycling between the extremities of deprivation and compensation.

For the Roman army, which consisted mostly of heavy infantry, foraging wasn't an easy task. Small groups of soldiers, who were sent to the fields to collect wheat crops, were often attacked by enemy cavalry units, which were quicker and faster than the Roman infantry. Supported by light-armed troops, the cavalry was important in the attack and defense of foraging parties. In order to avoid splitting the army into small vulnerable foraging units, Caesar established an "always-on-the-march" strategy with the view of getting his supplies more conveniently by moving camps to various places. Foraging and living off the land was practiced during spring and summer time, when crops were ripe. Winter was a bad time for an advancing army that depended on local food supplies; external food supplies were crucial during that season.

The Second and Third Macedonian Wars clearly illustrated the influence of food supply and seasonality on strategy, and vice versa. The Macedonian army moved into the mainland, where during the wintertime they forced the advanced Roman army to retreat as a result of problems with food supply. Winter was a bad time for war campaigns, and it still is today.

In the late Roman Empire (during Hadrian's reign), Roman soldiers cultivated and grew their own crops and vineyards. At that later time, the Roman army was mainly a defensive army. Not being on the move changed these soldier-warriors' routine to a more comfortable, less-aggressive phase. That may have been the first sign of the beginning of the end of the Roman Empire.

Summary

Macedonian, Spartan, and Roman warriors were always on the move. Army campaigns on foreign land forced these wandering warriors to adapt to different climates and seasons, and to adjust their diets accordingly. From an early age, they were trained to adapt to different daily, seasonal, and yearly natural cycles. Following the daily cycle, warriors cooked their own meals at night, and ate while camping. Cooking was popular among Romans. Emperors, army leaders, senators, historians and philosophers created their own recipes.

It's interesting to note that some wealthy people, like Cato or Cicero, were proud of the humble or "modest" meals they ate. It was their way of practicing austerity and sobriety. But in fact, these allegedly modest meals were beyond the reach of the poor.

Common people had to adjust rapidly to changes in conditions due to wars or natural disasters, such as famine or drought, since they depleted much of the available food supply. Because of constant dangers, insecurity, and life's hardships, the "nuclear family" predominated in the Greco-Roman world. Family members united together to help each other in times of crisis. Evening meals were dedicated to tightening the bonds of family and friends.

Roman men, soldiers, and civilians, had to adapt to a warrior way of life. Physical appearance was of crucial importance to these people; being in shape was a must. Therefore, they paid much attention to their diet, style of dress, and to physical activities.

The ideal "Warrior Diet" was supposed to supply the right nutrients for these active people so they could stay in shape and be strong enough to endure prolonged physical and mental pressure. The ideal Roman diet was based on a combination of all the food groups: vegetables, grains, oil, and legumes with meat, fish, eggs, or dairy. As mentioned, warriors who lived on vegetarian diets, based on grains and legumes only, did so because of shortages in the food supply. They preferred protein sources such as meat, cheese, or fish.

Vegetarian, high-grain diets often caused protein deficiencies, as well as mineral and vitamin malabsorption and deficiencies. Warriors were aware of that, and so they constantly looked for good sources of protein. Digestion and elimination were top priorities for ancient warriors. Fermented foods in the form of raw vinegar, fermented vegetables, fish, or wine, supplied these people with the friendly lactic-acid-producing bacteria and probiotics, essential for healthy digestive and metabolic systems.

As you've noticed, the diet kept by common people differed from that of the higher classes. Commoners and hard laborers often faced the threat of malnutrition or starvation, and therefore consumed whatever they could afford. Slaves, laborers, and poor people ate during the day. Noble men and soldiers who carried arms followed a diet that was based on a daily cycle—one meal

Applications to the Warrior Diet

Roman people considered themselves superior to their Greek slaves. Yet Greek slaves were in charge of educating and medically treating their Roman masters. Greek culture, wisdom, and mythology established the basic foundation of the Roman way of life. It's reasonable to conclude that the Roman diet, which consisted of mostly crudus (raw) food during the day, and warm, cooked meals at night, was in fact influenced by ancient Greek, Spartan, Athenian, and Macedonian traditions.

Romans, Spartans, and Macedonians were strong, tough people. Alexander the Great all but took over the world with a group of only 60,000 men. He conquered the Mediterranean, Middle East, and Egypt. He destroyed a whole Persian army and moved into India, where his army crossed 1,000 miles of desert by foot. This group of warriors was so potent that, man-for-man, they left more babies in their wake than any other advancing army in history. There are people today living in remote places throughout Asia, India, and Persia (now Iran) who still claim to be descendents of Alexander the Great.

The Spartans frequently demonstrated their courage and awesome might. At the pass of Thermopylae, three hundred Spartan warriors led by King Leonidas stopped a million-man Persian army under King Xerxes.

Roman warriors were notorious for their bravery. Julius Caesar destroyed a Gaul army that outnumbered the Romans two to one. As mentioned, the average Latin warrior was only 135-145 lbs. Yet he successfully fought face-to-face against a 180-lb. man from the north, whether a Gaul, a Celt, or a German.

Looking at Roman and Greek art, you can clearly see that the Roman and Greek warrior was lean and muscular. Julius Caesar was in his late fifties when he was assassinated, and at the time of his death was still lean and in good shape. The "lean 'n' mean" look of the warrior wasn't just an aesthetic concept. For an armed man who spent most of his life outdoors exercising and doing extreme physical activities— mobilizing heavy equipment from one place to another, at times marching thirty to forty miles a day and then engaging in face-to-face combat—the lean physique was a must.

Being as light and mighty as one could be was an essential factor for the survival of a warrior. Conversely, being heavy, slow, or sluggish could create a situation where one might not react quickly enough. For a warrior, that could be fatal. The lean look or —if you wish—the warrior's ideal body proportion was therefore more an issue of function than of fashion.

I have to say that being a soldier does not necessarily mean being in good shape. Army leaders like Napoleon, Czar Alexander of Russia, and Norman Schwartzkopf, for that matter, did not look lean or hard. That, of course, is just the physical look. But if you believe in "what you see is what you get," appearance has a lot to do with one's diet. My conclusion is that the ancient warrior diet of cycling between extremities of deprivation and compensation, with physical activities mostly during the day, was a major factor in shaping the characters of ancient warriors, as well as how they looked and the way they fought. Extreme deprivation, agitation, and anxiety during the day, and relaxation and compensation at night, made these warriors tough enough to endure pain and pressure for long periods, and still remain in good shape. Their Warrior Instinct kept them constantly alert to changes, and able to adapt quickly to different conditions.

The Warrior Diet was also followed by other ancient groups of warriors in different parts of the world. The common thread for all warriors was that they wandered. They moved from one place to another, living off the land—practically fighting their way as they went along.

The Ramadan holy fast of the Muslims (which is based on fasting during the day and eating only at night) mimics, in my opinion, the way that wild Arab warrior tribes lived in the sixth and seventh century in North Africa and the Middle East during Mohammad's time.

Steak Tartar is reminiscent of the way Mongolian warriors would tie meat to the back of their horses and ride until night, by which time the shaken and beaten meat had become soft and tender. Mongols were probably the most ferocious warriors in history. They were meat eaters—and the tradition of eating meat and milk is still popular among these nomadic people today. Mongolian warriors used to eat at night while camping. Their most nutritional food was mare (horse) milk, which is high in essential fatty acids

acids and is close in biological structure to human mother's milk. Mother's milk and colostrum were both popular among Greek and Roman physicians. They prescribed this dairy nectar to treat symptoms such as infections, headaches, or fever.

Conclusions

I've tried to relay the story of ancient warriors in the most objective, factual way. But how can anyone be completely objective? In my opinion, the Warrior Diet is an updated ancient diet. I think it would be impractical to follow an ancient diet without taking into account the changes that have occurred over time, and how these changes affect our lives today. Human nature hasn't changed much, but the world certainly has. Since we know much more today about the science of nutrition and its effects on the human body and mind, I was able to create a diet based on the old but with appropriate adjustments made for the twenty-first century. I truly believe that if Caesar were alive today, he'd follow a diet similar to the Warrior Diet.

In my opinion, a twenty-first century man or woman, who isn't involved in warrior activities, can still live like a warrior. As I've said before, cycling between undereating and overeating, detoxifying on a daily basis, exercising regularly, and naturally manipulating your hormones to a peak metabolic state, should trigger your Warrior Instinct.

Once triggered, this instinct will guide you to perform at your best both physically and mentally. I believe that with time you'll notice how your body naturally transforms itself while adapting to a warrior lifestyle. In other words, you'll become a warrior and look like one.

The Warrior Diet is actually a lesson from history. This diet is based on years of research, my own experience, as well as the experience of many others who have gone on it—and what I've offered here are my personal conclusions.

The Historical Role of Nutritional Carbohydrates—And Their Applications Today

Ancient warriors' high consumption of carbohydrates during campaigns may raise questions about the role carbs should play in diet. Whether this high-carb diet was an ideal warrior diet or not has already been discussed. However, the role carbohydrates play as a main source of nutrition is still an open issue today—and needs a fresh review.

Ever since Dr. Atkins' New Diet Revolution, The Zone, Protein Power Diet, and The Carbohydrate Addict's Diet hit bookstores and became bestsellers, carbs have become the "the Bad Guys on the Block." Millions of people today, who desperately wish to lose weight, try these low- or no-carb fad diets. And many of these dieters lose weight in the short run. Unfortunately, in the long run, many gain back more weight than they've lost. According to the low-carb diet concept, one will lose weight when carbs aren't available, because the body is forced to burn fat. That's the main trick. However, the issue of carbohydrates as a body fuel isn't so simple. The main argument made by low-carb diet gurus is that carbohydrates are not an essential nutrient food, and therefore one can live very well without them.

Let me offer some facts regarding the role of carbohydrates. They are:

Brain Fuel

The brain needs a mixed fuel of carbs, protein, and fat to function properly. Carbs are the main source of energy for the brain. Without a sufficient supply of carbs, you may feel anxious, dizzy, lethargic, or depressed. A mixed fuel works by activating different pleasure sensors in your brain. When there aren't enough carbs in the fuel, you may feel deprived and develop sugar cravings, which may in turn lead to compulsive bingeing.

Stress Blockers

Carbohydrates block cortisol (the stress hormone). The insulin hormone is a major cortisol blocker. That's one of the reasons people under stress tend to eat carbohydrate-rich foods. Moreover, without carbs, you may not be able to produce enough serotonin. Serotonin is a protein neurotransmitter in the brain, essential for feeling calm, relaxed, and happy.

Anti-aging

Serotonin is also the building block of the hormone melatonin. Without enough melatonin, you may suffer from sleep disorders and "chronic jet lag." Melatonin is a powerful antioxidant hormone, and is believed to possess some anticancerous and anti-aging properties. The older you get, the less melatonin is produced. Keeping your melatonin levels high, if nothing else, may help keep you young.

Clean Body Fuel

Carbohydrates are the cleanest fuel for energy. Your body breaks carbs into energy without any toxic byproducts. Conversely, when your body is forced to break protein and fat into energy, there will be toxic byproducts, such as ammonia, nitrates, free radicals or oxidized fatty acids—which will tax your system. Carbs are the most efficient fuel for energy. They metabolize faster than proteins and fats. By rapidly replenishing depleted glycogen reserves in muscle tissues and the liver, carbs spare muscle breakdown.

Metabolic Controllers

A daily supply of complex carbs will keep your thyroid level up. A healthy thyroid controls your body temperature, and keeps your metabolism intact.

Conclusions

You can see how chronic deprivation of carbohydrates in the long run may have some negative effects on your body and mind. Chronic carb-depletion, for prolonged periods of time, may eventually compromise your mood, your ability to relax, your metabolism, and may even accelerate the aging process. It probably sounds old-fashioned to recommend that people go back to eating carbs, especially today when low-carb diets are the darling of the media, as well as many celebrities, fashion models, and diet gurus.

The Warrior Diet is definitely not about carb-deprivation. In my opinion, the fact that warriors in the past were in such great shape had a lot to do with high-carb consumption. Eating carbs at night replenished these superactive men's bodies with clean fuel. It nourished them with specific essential nutrients, such as fibrous brans and certain phytonutrients that they could not get from any other food source. Most importantly, a supply of carbs at night was a major factor that fully completed the compensation effect of the diet. Since warriors lived under "fight or flight" conditions during the day—with all the agitation and anxiety that involved— they needed full compensation at night to calm down and give them a sense of pleasure and relaxation. I firmly believe that this compensation factor is what made these ancient warriors so capable of enduring intense physical and mental strain for such long periods of time.

My conclusions, therefore, are:

1. Without carbs there won't be complete compensation.

2. Only when the cycle of deprivation and compensation is complete can you benefit greatly from the Warrior Diet.

3. Diets based on chronic carb-deprivation will eventually leave you feeling constantly deprived and, in the long run, will fail.

The Warrior Diet isn't necessarily a high-carbohydrate diet. As you've seen in the "Overeating Phase," carbohydrates should be consumed during your evening meal—either with your cooked veggies and protein, or preferably after them if your goal is to lose body fat. In the latter case they should be the smallest component of your meal.

Different people have different needs. Competitive athletes and those involved in daily physical activities will need more carbs than weekend warriors will. Professional athletes who train twice a day, for example, may need to eat small snacks of carbs during the day, like ancient warriors did, to satisfy their high-calorie needs. People who burn thousands of calories during the day need to replenish their empty glycogen reserves to avoid muscle catabolism. However, since most people are not engaged in prolonged physical activities on a daily basis, the Warrior Diet generally eliminates carbs (except fruits and veggies) during the day. As noted earlier, you can cycle the diet according to your needs. In the "Warrior Diet Idea" I discuss how to cycle between days of high carbs and days of high protein. Use your instincts to choose the right cycle that will satisfy your needs.

In this discussion about nutritional carbohydrates, I refer to complex carbohydrates, preferably from whole foods such as rice, barley, oats, corn, potatoes, and yams. Sugar and other processed simple carbs should be minimized. They may have devastating effects on your body by overstimulating insulin, and may result in insulin insensitivity, food cravings, mood swings, and fat gain.

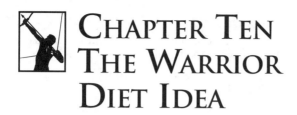

CHAPTER TEN
THE WARRIOR
DIET IDEA

The Warrior Diet, as I've said before, is not just a diet. It's a way of life. It is, as you know by now, based on triggering the Warrior Instinct through a daily cycle of undereating and overeating. Since this is a controversial diet, and goes against conventional rules, I feel it's important to discuss different ideas in relation to diet, nutrition, instincts, and a sense of freedom. I also question some conventional ideas or habits that, in my opinion, need to be re-evaluated.

Some ideas set forth here go beyond the diet, yet I believe will greatly benefit those who make the Warrior Diet a way of life.

Cycling the Warrior Diet

You can cycle the Warrior Diet in different ways: with days of undereating only, and other days where you choose to overeat. You can also alternate between days of high protein and others of high carbohydrates. However, if your goal is to lose body fat, high protein days are more effective.

There inevitably will be times when you're too busy, stressed, don't feel well, or may be romantically engaged and don't want to overeat. This is fine; you can undereat for a few days, and then resume your Warrior Diet routine. This is part of the leverage you have on this diet. Listen to your instincts. If you crave high carbs, you may need to satisfy calorie demands, or just calm down. Don't deny yourself any food group.

You can also go off the Warrior Diet, and then come back to it. This way you can practice the right diet for the right moment and always maintain the freedom to make choices. Some people choose to go off the Warrior Diet during holidays or on weekends, to enjoy eating meals both during the day and evening with family or friends. This is okay. You should be able to live with the Warrior Diet, without feeling deprived.

• Going Off the Warrior Diet

As mentioned, you may choose to go off the Warrior Diet on some days, or for a short while. Let's say you go on a trip, or are not cooking and want to enjoy eating small meals throughout the day. This is fine.

Every time I've been on trips and gone off the Warrior Diet, my meals are more frequent but smaller, and I lose weight. This is probably because my body's metabolism has been accelerated by the practice of overeating. If you choose to go off the Warrior Diet, and have small meals throughout the day, for a short while your body will likely burn more than you actually eat. This heightened metabolism will remain for a while; however, if you go off the Warrior Diet completely and return to a routine of eating a few small meals per day, *I believe your body will readjust to a lower metabolic rate.* It's my contention that once you've practiced the Warrior Diet for a time, and have experienced its incredible benefits, you'll eventually come back to it because it's so effective.

• How Often Can You Deviate from the Warrior Diet?

You can deviate as often as you want, but my assumption is that you won't want to. Freedom is the most important thing, so do whatever you want. Use your instincts.

Wild cats look their best when they're hungry. So do you.

• What Makes You Stay on the Warrior Diet?

The Warrior Diet is so powerful that it's like a gravitational pull, bringing you back because you'll feel great when practicing it. This is partly due to something that happens during undereating, what I call the "brain-power factor" or "opening the brain barrier." This holds especially true for those who like to feel highly energetic, alert, clear-minded, focused, and want to boost their creative or competitive drive.

There's something like a switch that's turned on after you adapt to undereating, and you become almost addicted to this "crispness" of your brain. Who wouldn't enjoy the "high" feeling that the Undereating Phase provides?

During the Undereating Phase, physical hunger can be turned into spiritual hunger. Many people have long believed that one can only experience a deep spiritual awareness when fasting. This said, I should reiterate the full satisfaction and sense of freedom that you can achieve every day during the Overeating Phase, when you can eat as much as you want with no guilt involved, and will pleasantly calm down. Every day has a happy end.

Once you experience the Warrior Diet, you should feel an awakening of a deep, deep instinct. Imagine people who've never had sex, and then suddenly do—and it's great. Would they want to give it up? I truly believe this diet is so strong that you won't let it go. Once your Warrior Instinct is triggered, no one can take it away from you. It would be like trying to extract raw meat from a tiger's jaws.

Cycling the Autonomic Nervous System (The Acid-Base Cycle)

The Warrior Diet is the only diet I'm aware of that achieves the correct balance between the two parts of the ANS (the autonomic nervous system), the sympathetic, and parasympathetic systems. The sympathetic nervous system (SNS) is responsible for all "fight or flight" reactions, and usually works in an acidic environment. It's mainly catabolic. The parasympathetic nervous system, on the other hand, is responsible for digestion and elimination, and usually works in an alkaline environment. It's mainly anabolic. These two systems are somehow antagonistic when activated simultaneously.

Many people who eat frequent meals during the day, and are often under stress, suffer from digestive problems, lethargy, or exhaustion. These problems can occur because the adrenal "fight or flight" system contradicts the digestion and elimination system. On the contrary, the Warrior Diet alternates between the sympathetic and parasympathetic systems. During the day the sympathetic system activates your alertness and ability to handle stress (the "fight or flight" reactions). By the time you reach the Overeating Phase you've already consumed living foods (fruits, vegetables, and juices made from them), so your body is alkalized. Alkalizing your body will reduce the catabolic-acidic effect of the SNS, and prepare you for the parasympathetic system of digestion and elimination. The Warrior Diet is the only diet I'm aware of that uses both systems without compromising one or the other.

The Instinct to Overeat

Many practitioners and diet gurus tell us not to overeat and support this with reasons like, "It places too much pressure on the body" and "it creates an imbalance." Yet people do overeat, and when they do they usually feel guilty. Well, I'm going to be the first one to say that overeating can be good for you—moreover, that doing so is instinctual. And, like any primal instinct you try to repress and shove inside, it'll come up anyway.

• The Overeating Syndrome (Deprivation Leads to Uncontrolled Bingeing)

Overeating is an instinctual way for the body to compensate when it's chronically underfed, malnourished, starving, emotionally or mentally deprived. The urge to overeat can also be triggered when the body tries to pick up its metabolism, which may have declined as a result of prolonged low-calorie diets. Overeating can work for you if you control it—by inducing it at the right time. This is discussed extensively in the "Overeating" chapter.

If you don't let your body overeat when it needs to, it's going to haunt you. For instance, many people go to the fridge late at night, open it, and start bingeing. When you ask them why they do this, they often say it's almost like a demonic force making them binge, and they can't stop themselves. A fair number of people binge compulsively. I believe that a large percentage of bingers do so because they feel they are deprived. Deprivation is a key factor in uncontrolled bingeing. The real question is whether bingeing is controlled or uncontrolled. When people are out of balance, or feel deprived—due to unhealthy diets and eating habits—they often develop chronic food cravings, which, in turn, lead to compulsive, uncontrolled bingeing. Bingeing under these circumstances is obviously not a good thing.

• Overeating Boosts Metabolism—Your metabolism is as good as your last meal

One of the most important benefits of overeating on the Warrior Diet is that you boost your metabolism. Mainstream thought regarding metabolism is that you're as good as the calories you eat per day. Some theories say that if you want to lose weight, you just have to reduce your calories. Usually this works, up to a certain point. But after a week or two, the body's metabolism slows down, so you have to maintain this lower level of calories or continue reducing them to keep the weight off—then if you eat even just an extra tomato, you may gain weight. Of course I'm teasing about the tomato, but you get the point.

Why would your metabolism slow down so much? Because when you decrease your calories, the body, through adaptation, attempts to maintain itself at this new lower level in order to survive. So, if all of a sudden you increase the calories—you may gain weight. That's what happens to body builders. In-season, body builders look lean because of strict calorie reductions. Off-season, they usually gain weight, often quite suddenly.

I believe the best way to lose body fat without the above side effect is to reduce calories for a few days, then increase them somewhat, in order not to let the body adapt to the low-calorie diet. On the Warrior Diet, you go through this process practically every day, cycling between undereating and overeating.

As mentioned above, most nutritionists and dieticians say that what counts are the calories consumed per day, however, I believe it's the calories per meal. Or, to say it differently, it's the amount of food/intensity of the meal that counts. This theory also applies to workouts. We already know that you can exercise moderately for three hours without making progress. Yet, a ten-minute intense workout can be effective enough to stimulate muscle development and strength. So, it's often the intensity that forces your body to adapt, not necessarily the length or the volume.

When you divide your meals into three-to-six per day, like most typical diets suggest, and each meal is approximately 150 to 300 calories, that's what the body remembers, the consumption of 150–300 calories per meal. The Warrior Diet's concept is different. It's built on intensity. So when you consume, for instance, 1,000-1,500 calories in a meal, that's what the body remembers. There's a hormonal acceleration that occurs with such intense meals; the body tries to increase its metabolism in accordance with the big meal you ate.

Recent scientific experiments conducted on mice show that mice fasting for eighteen hours, without being overfed, suffered from low thyroid and slow metabolism. However, mice that were overfed, and then went through an 18-hour fast, kept their thyroid hormone at a normal level and their metabolism high.

I believe that those who undereat and overeat will gradually increase their metabolism.

• How Many Calories Should You Consume during the Overeating Phase?

For some people overeating will be 600 calories a meal. For others, like myself, it's 1,500–3,000 calories a meal. Building up must be done gradually. Don't jump to 3,000 calories per meal too quickly.

Once you begin to practice the Warrior Diet, you'll find that your metabolism gradually picks up to the point that when everybody else gains weight during the holidays, which involves big meals, you won't because you eat like this every day. What people call overeating during the holidays is actually an average meal for a warrior.

Glycogen Stretching: To Boost Metabolism, Build Muscles, and Lose Body Fat

Glycogen is the carbohydrate energy-reserve in our muscles and liver. For sedentary people, glycogen supplies only a few hundred calories. After these available calories are burned, they may experience some unpleasant symptoms, such as dizziness, nervousness, or exhaustion. Conversely, a trained person will be able to burn twice as many glycogen-available calories without side effects. Maintaining a proper diet and exercise routine can increase glycogen reserves and endurance.

Let me explain "training to stretch glycogen reserves." Let's say that you workout like a warrior, on an empty stomach, and then overeat. After a few months, you may succeed to increase the glycogen reserves in your muscles by simply depleting and then overcompensating carbs on a daily basis. So your body gradually adapts by increasing its own glycogen reserves.

Glycogen holds water in the muscle tissue. That's what gives your muscle a "pumped" look. When people are depleted of glycogen, it looks like they've shrunk but they haven't lost muscle, they've lost glycogen. Replenishing empty glycogen reserves by overeating will give the muscle back its pumped look. The more you delete and pump, the more the adaptation process will lead to what I call "glycogen stretching."

The method of carb depletion and then carb loading is popular among endurance athletes. Those who try it say it gives them huge increases in stamina, to endure prolonged physical strain.

How Much Body Fat Should You Have?

There are a lot of myths out there. I believe excessive fat storage is unnecessary, because fat in any living creature is a storage house for toxins in your body. It's also a factor in producing estrogen. On top of all this, it's believed that obesity is correlated with insulin insensitivity and diabetes. So, a "bulge" isn't good for you. After a certain minimum amount of fat, you don't need any more. Ideally, adult males should have no more than 10 percent body fat. However, people have different genetic predispositions for body fat. Therefore, optimum body fat levels differ slightly from one person to the next.

Some contend that fat tissues are necessary for you because they're thermogenic, and give you warmth. I believe this is a wrong assumption. In my opinion, there's no correlation between fat and heat. Body heat depends on your metabolism; how efficiently you burn energy through your glandular, hormonal, and cellular systems is what effects body heat.

Building Muscles Without Gaining Fat

You can build muscles and not gain fat if you eat the way I suggest. If you consume a large amount of protein, the correct mineral supplements and enough carbohydrates (preferably complex carbs) to moderately boost insulin, you create an anabolic environment. Moreover, I believe the body's ability to utilize protein can increase by twofold after undereating. Once you're depleted, you reach the potential to be your best when you do eat—and can accelerate the anabolic process of building muscles without gaining fat.

As long as you keep the Warrior Diet rules of eating, and gradually increase the amount of protein per meal, you can accelerate muscle gain. From my personal experience, the amount of protein you eat will eventually determine how you build muscle tissues. Whenever you ingest 2g of protein per pound of body weight, you stimulate a natural anabolic process. As long as you have the carbs at the end of the meal, and as the smallest component, you'll gain muscle without gaining body fat.

Insulin Insensitivity

Many people suffer from insulin insensitivity. As a result of this, they often convert carbohydrates into triglycerides, which leads to high cholesterol, water retention, weight gain, hyperglycemia, and prediabetes. People develop insulin insensitivity as a result of eating sweets and overly processed carbohydrate foods throughout the day. Other reasons for developing it are due to overconsumption of bad fats or deficiencies of essential fats, especially omega-3. Consequently, the pancreas becomes overtaxed by the continual oversecretion of insulin and pancreatic enzymes, which desperately work to break down the carbs and remove glucose from the blood to avoid raising blood sugar.

Eating frequent meals throughout the day doesn't leave the body enough time to recuperate. Over time the insulin receptors become insensitive, and so the body secretes even more insulin in order to reduce blood sugar. This leads to high fluctuations of blood sugar, and one may feel hungrier as a result, and so eat even more carbohydrates. If this vicious cycle continues unabated, one eventually gains weight and becomes sick.

Conversely, after you've gone through the Undereating Phase of the Warrior Diet, you are at peak hormonal and enzymatic levels. By stabilizing your insulin, you manipulate it/this hormone to work as an anabolic agent, which builds lean muscle tissue. You'll also be able to metabolize carbs into energy without blood-sugar fluctuations. Stabilized insulin is a key to antiaging and health.

The Sense of Freedom

I'd like to discuss what freedom and the sense of freedom mean, what happens when people are deprived of it, and what happens when they have it. I'll also offer my perspective on how freedom relates to negative emotions, such as anger, fear, anxiety, and pain, and how it relates to positive feelings such as relief, happiness, excitement, and joy.

Freedom is an ideal. Nobody is completely free. But *we experience a sense of freedom when we feel that we have the ability to make choices and satisfy our primal instincts.*

This is the only diet I'm aware of that doesn't limit your sense of freedom. Once you find your own healthy cycle, you'll feel free because you're in control, your body is rejuvenating again and again, and when you eat, you eat what your body craves. You'll enjoy your meals and will stop eating when you want to, not because your ego, or guilt, or others tell you to. This is quite a difference from other diets.

On the Warrior Diet, you'll likely accelerate your metabolism and lose body fat. In earlier chapters I discussed how during the Undereating Phase, and especially when you exercise on an empty stomach, your growth hormone is boosted, and while you switch to the glucagon system, you're ensured of hours of fat-burning on a daily basis. Most of your energy during the day actually comes from burning fat. Just think how exhilarating it'll be to realize that by following the right cycle your body will naturally transform itself and become leaner and stronger!

• How a "Sense of Freedom" Relates to Your Diet

Instincts create desires. Every time you satisfy a desire that derives from a deep instinct, such as creative, sexual, or aggressive ones, you feel pleasure and a sense of freedom. People generally fantasize about things when they're deprived of them. A funny example of this is Kurt Vonnegut's book *Breakfast of Champions,* where people go to the movies to watch other people on the screen eating cheesecake. In this futuristic comedy, eating cheesecake is outlawed. His satire points out how sick we've become.

You may ask, "If I actually fulfill all my fantasies and instincts, does that mean I won't have any others?" Far from it. You'll have greater fantasies—more romantic, more adventurous, more creative, and more spiritual ones. You may take more chances and more risks, such as launch a new business, help the less fortunate, or work in some way to improve your life. In short, you'll become more ambitious and successful in whatever you choose to do because you're not stuck in primitive fantasies like eating cheesecake. Most importantly, when you satisfy your desires, you gain in feelings of pleasure. Without pleasure, you'll feel deprived and miserable. Life is too short to not get the best from it.

The Romantic Instinct— A New Definition for Romanticism

What does romantic mean? What makes someone a "romantic?" What is a romantic act? Romantic instinct? Romantic aspect?

Romantic period? Since these words and phrases, although used for a long time, aren't always clearly defined, I think they need some clarification.

I'm aware that what I am about to say is debatable, so take it any way you want. You may agree with me, and you may not.

It's my strong belief that romanticism is based on an instinct that's related to and comes from the same source as the "Warrior Instinct." The romantic instinct is a primal instinct that identifies a person's uniqueness, makes him question rules, and fight to keep his integrity intact.

The core of romanticism is the concept of breaking an established rule in order to build a new one. And a romantic act is the action of doing just that. For example, the story of *Romeo and Juliet* is romantic because of their struggle to build a relationship in spite of their family's rules. *Romeo and Juliet* are romantic heroes. Seeking each other out in spite of their families was a romantic act, and killing themselves made it even more romantic. Sacrificing one's own life because of love goes against the rule— or instinct— to survive. Throughout history, a romantic aura has surrounded those who were ready to sacrifice their lives for a cause they believed in strongly.

A romantic aspect can emerge solely by breaking a rule. Criminals, whores, and antiheroes, for instance, who defy and break societal rules have often been the subjects of literary giants, like Balzac and Dostoyevsky. Outlaws like Jesse James, Billy the Kid, Butch Cassidy, and Bonnie and Clyde, are considered romantic heroes mainly because they broke the rules.

As noted, romanticism is based on an instinct. Children, for example, have an innate and very fresh romantic instinct. When an authority figure, like a parent or teacher, tells a young child to do (or not to do) something, they often try to disobey. It's also very common for children to joke about their teachers. Kids have a great sense of humor, and humor by itself involves breaking rules. I truly believe that it's the romantic instinct deep within our subconscious that makes us enjoy jokes that break taboos, and the child within us that cracks up when we hear or see something funny. Children's romantic instincts, unfortunately, are often crushed over time, since they seek approval and are inevitably faced with so many parental, religious, political, and societal rules that they begin to feel guilty when they go against them. Nevertheless, these primal romantic desires and instincts still lie deep within us. I believe that every romantic story, in literature and in life, somehow involves triggering this instinct.

To "keep order," society places many taboos that are antiromantic. This is understandable since if everyone were romantic, it would be impossible to maintain control. But when this primal instinct is controlled and inhibited, like anything that's inhibited, there are side effects and symptoms, such as feelings of frustration, anger, deprivation, lack of freedom, and boredom.

We're living in a world where false romanticism abounds. There isn't enough space here to fully philosophize about this subject, so let me just say that any seemingly romantic idea that appeals to a crowd of people is probably falsely romantic. True romanticism is individualistic and endorses uniqueness. I'm not suggesting that people break rules or laws. However, I am saying that the ability to instinctively question rules is necessary when you want to improve upon something, make a change, or create something new.

How This Relates to the Warrior Diet

As noted, I believe that the "Warrior Instinct" manifests itself through the romantic instinct. By triggering the "Warrior Instinct," you'll become more romantic, you'll instinctively identify your uniqueness, and you will be ready to take action as needed to keep it intact.

False vs. True Romanticism

What I call false romanticism is the most common variety. As an example, if you were raised to be civilized, peaceful, and respectful of other people's lives, and then suddenly your country declares war and tells you to go and fight and kill, this may sound very romantic. Being a soldier does in fact have a romantic aspect to it, since it implies the readiness to sacrifice your life for a cause.

However, going to war with all its seemingly "romantic" aspects didn't come from you; it came from the establishment and, therefore, to me it's false. Conversely, if you *volunteer* to go and fight and help a cause, then you're doing something that's truly romantic, since you initiated it and are following your personal beliefs while keeping your integrity intact.

Romantic rituals and holidays, like weddings and Valentine's Day, are other examples that I believe have little to do with real romanticism. People mistakenly confuse rituals celebrating mating with the truly romantic act of falling in love. When a man falls in love, for instance, his romantic instinct kicks in and he becomes a "romantic fool," meaning he'd do things that are out of the ordinary, like sacrifice his time and money, just to be with, and satisfy, his loved one. Unfortunately, after some time, many married couples no longer act romantically. Their marriages become routine, and the only romantic things left are the so-called "celebrations of love," holidays like Valentine's Day and wedding anniversaries.

This said, there are people who are constantly romantic, break routines, and continue to fall in love with their mates.

Following stiff routines is the antithesis of romanticism. Breaking routines are like breaking rules. When the romantic instinct is triggered, people are instinctively more adventurous, more creative, and are ready to take more risks.

In the matter of love and relationships, I truly believe that once this romantic instinct is unleashed, it'll instinctively guide you to act romantically at all times. When this instinct kicks in, a person is in their best shape to attract their mate. Falling in love, with the desire to give to, share with, and protect someone is based on an instinctual drive that involves a lot of changes. Being with someone and having a family together demands more responsibilities and an ability to handle all the changes necessary to that union. As I've said before, it's the romantic instinct that encourages you to go through all these changes and continue to care for someone else while creating new lives.

You may ask "Can you be a romantic or do a romantic act without breaking a rule?" My answer to this is no. All romantic acts involve breaking rules or routines, and doing things out of the ordinary. Being romantic extends beyond love, relationships, and the breaking of old habits. It is romantic to make a new resolution and create something new. It is romantic to be brave enough to stand up for your rights—or someone else's rights—and be ready to face the consequences. As I've said, true romanticism comes from deep inside you. When you commit a romantic act and go against the rules or routines, you're actually fighting to keep your integrity and uniqueness intact. This, in my opinion, is what makes the romantic instinct a manifestation of the "Warrior Instinct."

The Aggressive Instinct

In his controversial book *On Aggression*, anthropologist Desmond Morris tries to prove that aggression is a primal instinct necessary for survival. Aggression doesn't need to be expressed through violence. In a way, violence is a result of suppressed aggression. Once it explodes, it goes out of control. Aggression has its positive side. It manifests itself through competitive drive, as a potential force needed for self-defense, and for expanding one's territory.

This is a major subject, which deserves more space. For now, I'd like to say that I truly feel that aggression is indeed a primal instinct with both bad and good sides, and it should be thought of accordingly. Aggression is essential for survival. Without it, you'll either end up a saint, or just plain old dead.

The Myth of Eating Whole Foods Only

Christian Scientists, and some holistic health gurus, believe that you should eat only whole foods. They say taking supplements may knock you out of balance. I understand where they're coming from, since whole foods, especially raw foods, should supply all your essential nutrients. However, we don't live in a pristine world. Conditions today, like environmental pollutants, are big problems. Therefore, I feel some supplementation is often necessary to make up for the lost nutrients that existed in greater quantities in food in the past. However, I also believe there's a need for an alternative to the commercial, synthetic powders people take today. Ideally, nutritional supplements should be derived from whole, live food, and should be taken like food.

Chemical and Environmental Toxins— and Other Stressors in Everyday Life

Most diet books start with lots of current statistics of the frightening increase in obesity in the last half of the twentieth century. Many people today are aware of these stats, and so go on this or that diet. One doesn't have to be a rocket scientist to figure out the important role diet plays in our health, and the link between obesity and heart disease, diabetes, arthritis, and other degenerative diseases, including cancer.

But what many people don't know is that other factors—some of which are environmental, may contribute to the way people look, feel, and what they suffer from today.

Chemical factors, like petroleum-based pesticides, herbicides, and fertilizers, hormones and antibiotics in the meats, poultry, milk, and eggs we buy in the grocery store, environmental toxins like DDT, estrogenic plastic derivatives, and oral contraceptives in our water supply, and contaminants in the fish we eat—these are all examples of what I call "Stealth Factors." On a daily basis, we don't realize (and can't feel) that these toxic factors are present. There's nothing more dangerous than stealth toxins coupled with ignorance—because the inability to see or feel these dangers makes us even more vulnerable.

Data shows how destructive these (mainly man-made) forces are. Food additives, like nitrates or nitrites, pesticides, herbicides, hormones, antibiotics, estrogenic derivatives, plastic derivatives, and DDT are some of the major catalysts for a wide spectrum of modern diseases, ones that barely existed in the past. The National Cancer Institute found an increased risk of leukemia in children whose parents used pesticides in their garden or home. Another disorder that's been linked to food additives and chemical preservatives is Attention Deficit Disorder (ADD). Moreover, antibiotic residues found in non-organic meat and dairy leads to new mutations of antibiotic-resistant bacteria that may cause new infections (or infectious diseases), which are resistant to antibiotic drugs.

Of even more concern are the plastic derivatives, pesticides, and estrogenic-like chemicals in our food supply. These toxins have been connected to male sterility and the increase in cancer rates. Male sterility today is higher than ever, and other unpleasant estrogenic effects, like "stubborn fat" and the "feminization" of men abound. According to the American Chemical Society, sperm count in men worldwide is 50% lower than it was 50 years ago. And, according to the same source, young male alligators in pesticide-contaminated lakes in Florida have such small penises they're unable to function sexually.

Farmers have been found to have a relatively high incidence of some cancers, including multiple meyloma (cancer of the bones), lymphomas, skin melanomas, leukemia, and cancer of the lip, stomach, prostate, and brain. Work-related exposure to chemicals was theorized to be causing them.

People with estrogen-related diseases, such as breast cancer and prostate cancer are at all-time highs. According to an American Chemical Society report, the incidence of prostate cancer has doubled in the past fifty years. And, while the incidence of breast cancer was one in twenty in 1960, it increased to one in nine in 1998. Since 1978, Israel banned three estrogenic pesticides: Lindane, DDT, and BHC. By 1986 the death rate from breast cancer among Israeli women below the age of 44 had dropped by 30%. Conversely, breast cancer rates among women who live in other industrialized countries have skyrocketed.

Steroid hormones in our meat and dairy can have devastating effects on everyone, especially children and infants. Premature puberty and child mortality have been linked to the hormones in non-organic meats and milk. These are only some of the consequences of chemical stealth toxins in the food and water supply.

The most dangerous of all stealth factors is radiation. I'm not just referring to nuclear radiation. We live in a world today that is overradiated and, as a result, are exposed nonstop to "slow radiation" that, put simply, is slowly killing us. Radioactive minerals penetrate the human food chain and cause different kinds of malignant cancers. These toxic materials aren't cycled like other organic materials.

For instance, the life expectancy of iodine 131 is about 160 years. Once this radioactive iodine penetrates the body, it occupies the place of the natural organic iodine mineral, which severely damages the body's metabolic process. Iodine 131 may be the main reason for cancer of the thyroid gland.

Some radioactive isotopes, like strontium 90 have a life expectancy of 360 years. Once a radioactive mineral penetrates the body, it binds to the organ that needs this mineral most and creates a chain reaction that causes catastrophic damage. I can go on and on, but let's just say that all of these stealth factors are extremely dangerous to one's health—and not knowing about them leaves us completely defenseless.

As mentioned, those most in danger are infants, children, and the elderly. Infants' and children's' immune systems are not fully developed, and since they have such small bodies, pound for pound, the toxic effect is much greater on them than on adults. The elderly often suffer from age-related, compromised immune systems, so toxins have an accelerated effect on them.

It seems there is nowhere to run. *But*—and this is a big but—the good news is that there is, in fact, a lot that we can do to defend ourselves against these stealth factors. I cover practical ways to enable you to defend yourself from stealth factors throughout this book: through diet, proper nutrition, and getting on the "Warrior Cycle." I also talk about ways to remove toxins from the body through different methods of detoxification.

I discuss several ways to help protect against the effects of environmental toxins next.

Protecting Yourself Against Environmental Toxins

• The First Defense Against Radioactive, Environmental Toxins

The first defense against environmental toxins, such as radiation, is saturating your body with minerals. Once cellular mineral saturation occurs, there's less possibility for the radioactive minerals to be absorbed into your body's organs. The best way to ensure mineral saturation is by following a daily detoxification routine, in which you ingest live fruits, as well as freshly prepared fruit and vegetable juices during the day. Besides supplying the body with live minerals, fruits and veggie juices are high in antioxidant nutrients and live enzymes, which defend the body against the free radicals created by radiation exposure. Moreover, alkalizing the system will strengthen your body's resistance to radioactive stressors.

As you can see, the Warrior Diet will give you a first protection against environmental radiation. Radioactive fallout is everywhere; therefore, the danger of being exposed to radioactive minerals is constant. Daily detoxification and mineral saturation is the first defense.

There are also certain foods and herbs that have within them special properties to protect the body from environmental radiation. These foods and herbs contain certain nutrient and mineral complexes that create a natural process of chelation. Chelation occurs when a nutrient pulls out, or neutralizes, toxins and radioactive materials that penetrate the system.

Following is a list of foods, nutrients, and herbs that have antiradiation properties:

Antiradiation Foods, Nutrients, and Herbs

Foods and Nutrients:

Sea Vegetables—Kelp, arame, kombu, and hijiki are all high in sodium alginate, which is the best chelator for pulling radioactive toxins from the body.

Miso—is high in minerals and is a strong alkalizer, which is believed to protect the body against radioactive minerals.

Beet Juice—is known as a liver and blood detoxifier. Beets are high in organic iron, which protects the body from plutonium and radioactive iron.

Super Foods:
Bee Pollen, Blue-Green Algae, High-Sulfur Vegetables

• *Bee Pollen*—Is high in minerals, vitamins, and live enzymes. Pound-for-pound, bee pollen is the highest protein food, higher than meat or dairy. Clinically, bee pollen has been shown to significantly reduce the side effects of chemotherapy. Bee pollen is also high in lecithin, which helps protect the nervous system. It's also high in nucleic acids, which protects the system from radioactive exposure.

• *Blue-Green Algae*—The high content of minerals, chlorophyll, and antioxidant nutrients in blue-green algae make this super food a great antiradiation supplement.

• *High-Sulfur Protein-Containing Vegetables*—Broccoli, cabbage, cauliflower, kale, Brussels sprouts, garlic, and onions are all high in the antioxidant sulfur-containing protein cysteine. Cysteine neutralizes free radicals, and protects against x-rays as well as radioactive minerals such as cobalt and sulfur.

Fiber: Vegetable, Grain, Legume, Seed and Fruit Fibers

Fiber helps to chelate radioactive material out of the system, including fibers containing phytates (which are found in grains and legumes), and pectin, a soluble fiber found in fruits and seeds. Lignans, which are in flaxseeds, have also been shown to possess great chelation properties.

High-Chlorophyll Foods: Leafy, Green Vegetables, Spirulina, Chlorella, Grass Sprouts, Parsley

Consuming high-chlorophyll foods, such as parsley, leafy greens, spirulina, and chlorella helps to significantly reduce the effects of radiation. The high-enzyme content of grass sprouts aids in detoxifying and neutralizing free radicals.

> As a general rule, peeling fruits and vegetables reduces the danger of exposure to radioactive fallout toxins.

Herbs: Siberian Ginseng, Astragalus, Echinacea

• *Siberian Ginseng*—is an adaptogenic herb. It's been found to rebalance and heal the body from physiological, emotional, and environmental stresses. Siberian Ginseng is one of the best herbs to combat the dangers associated with environmental radiation, x-ray exposure, and chemotherapy.

• *Astragalus*—boosts the immune system and thus helps to defend the system against radiation.

• *Echinacea/Goldenseal*—Echinacea is an immune booster and blood purifier. Goldenseal, besides being a potent immune booster, is believed to carry some anticancerous properties. Combining echinacea with goldenseal, in my opinion, works better than echinacea alone, particularly when you're sick. Pregnant or lactating women should consult their physician before taking them.

The best way to take these herbs is to cycle their supplementation on a few weeks-on, few weeks-off basis.

Note:

Some of the foods listed, such as fruits, freshly prepared fruit and veggie juices, bee pollen, and blue-green algae are best taken during the day on an empty stomach. Doing so will accelerate the detoxification effect, and assimilation of their essential nutrients. All the other foods and herbs listed can be ingested at any time of the day, or with your evening meal.

Warrior Greens is a nutritional supplement designed to help protect against environmental radiation. It's a proprietary blend of organic live grass with wildly grown blue-green algae, chlorella, and noni from India. Warrior Greens are processed to keep all life forces within the product. It's high in all vital nutrients and enzymes, which are essential for detoxification, digestion, and overall health. For more on this, see the "Warrior Nutritional Supplements" chapter

Prostate Enlargement Related Problems

Many men, who are understandably concerned about prostate cancer, ask whether there is anything they can do to reduce their odds of contracting it. What follows is my personal opinion and is not meant to suggest or guarantee that it is a cure for those that already suffer from prostate enlargement-related problems.

The most common opinions today about prostate cancer is that it's "accidentally" contracted due to a genetic predisposition. The current consensus in the mainstream medical community is that dehydro-testosterone (DHT), the so-called "bad testosterone," is what causes prostate cancer. DHT is a derivative of testosterone that binds to the androgen receptors inside the prostate gland, and is believed to be what makes the cells proliferate and become cancerous. This may be true, but I strongly believe it's not the whole truth.

In fact, I question this theory outright. Aging is correlated with lower testosterone production. Moreover, aging accelerates the conversion of testosterone into estrogen. So, if the DHT or oversecretion of testosterone causes prostate cancer, why are the majority of men who have it elderly, and have already lost quite a bit of their testosterone?

In my opinion, a combination of factors, such as estrogen, DHT, the so-called "bad testosterone," prolactin, and age-related high cholesterol may be what really creates enlargement of the prostate, or prostate cancer. More and more studies show that prolonged abuse of certain chemicals, exposure to pesticides, excessive alcohol consumption, and an unhealthy diet may all create a situation where your body becomes loaded with estrogenic substances. This could, in turn, have an estrogenic effect on your prostate. I feel it's this phenomenon, coupled with an estrogen imbalance, or the inability of the liver to detoxify estrogenic substances or derivatives, which may eventually accelerate prostate enlargement.

Prolactin (the hormone that produces milk) is also correlated with prostate enlargement-related diseases. Prolactin accelerates the penetration of testosterone to the prostate gland and its conversion into DHT inside the prostate gland. It's this conversion to DHT that makes the cells proliferate and causes the enlargement of the prostate. Elevation of prolactin can be due to a complex set of factors, including having a low thyroid and aging.

DHT Can Work for You

DHT is not always the bad guy. DHT is the most potent testosterone derivative, which positively affects potency. Moreover, DHT cannot penetrate the prostate gland from the blood. Only free testosterone (testosterone that is not bound to GHGB—gonadal hormone-binding globulins) can penetrate the prostate gland Only once it's then inside may it convert into DHT, and then, with estrogen or prolactin, possibly cause prostate enlargement, or even cancer. Drugs such as Proscar and Propecia work to reduce blood DHT and therefore to alleviate prostate enlargement symptoms (Proscar) and protect against hair loss (Propecia). However, both Proscar and Propecia have side effects, including impotence. So, following this line of thinking, the question is: What happens when blood DHT is increased?

Stay with me now. In an absurd way, by increasing blood DHT, testosterone levels decline. Therefore, the less testosterone penetrates the prostate, the less DHT is produced inside the gland and, as a result, symptoms and damage may be reduced, or even cleared.

The Warrior Diet as First Defense Against Prostate-Related Problems

I believe the Warrior Diet may help prevent prostate cancer since the long, daily period of undereating (controlled fasting) helps the liver detoxify all these chemicals and estrogenic derivatives. Ingesting live (raw) fruits and vegetables on a daily basis, which are loaded with live nutrients, helps the liver detoxify for much of each day.

If you don't tax the liver by consuming frequent meals, more energy is saved for digestion and elimination. Eating three to six meals a day may exhaust the liver's enzyme pool, and may eventually lead to liver congestion and toxification, which compromises this organ's ability to do its essential job. A congested or toxic liver cannot effectively handle all the food you eat, or break down and eliminate enough toxins. Estrogenic derivatives can then infect the blood and cause all these ill effects.

As I've said again and again, practicing the Undereating Phase (controlled fasting) on a daily basis is possibly the most important element of the Warrior Diet, and is one of the main reasons it's so powerful.

Avoiding estrogenic foods and chemicals (see list) further helps the liver to detoxify. Finally, eating the foods I suggest in this book, and taking the right nutritional supplements, enables you to ingest the nutrients to help protect against the effects of estrogen— while manipulating your hormonal balance to reach maximum metabolic efficiency.

To sum up, if you detoxify daily, eat the foods recommended, and minimize consumption of estrogenic foods and substances, I believe you will stand a far greater chance of keeping yourself healthy and avoiding prostate problems.

Estrogenic Foods and Substances (to Avoid):

- *All meat that is not organic (due to the estrogen hormones inside), such as red meat, chicken, turkey, lamb, pork*

- *All dairy and dairy products that are not organic, due to the estrogen and prolactin hormones inside*
- *Petroleum-based pesticides, herbicides, fertilizers, which are found in non-organic produce*
- *Wheat gluten (those who are sensitive to wheat)*
- *Soy oil (those who are sensitive to soy)*
- *Alcohol*
- *Marijuana*

Natural Supplements Help Alleviate Prostate Enlargement Related Symptoms

Pygeum Bark and Saw Palmetto

Pygeum Bark and Saw Palmetto berries are natural supplements that have been used traditionally to alleviate symptoms of Benign Prostate Hyperplasia (BPH).

Pygeum

Pygeum is an evergreen African tree. The bark of the trunk is the part of the tree that is used for medicinal purposes. It is often mixed with palm oil or milk.

It's interesting to note that certain substances in pygeum, such as n-docosanol (a triterpene), significantly reduces serum prolactin levels. As noted, prolactin increases the uptake of testosterone and increases the conversion to dihydrotestosterone (DHT) inside the prostate gland. Clinical trials and numerous studies support the fact that pygeum effectively reduces the symptoms of BPH

Fertility—Pygeum may improve infertility-related problems in men who suffer from diminished prostatic secretion. Pygeum helps to increase prostatic secretion and improve seminal fluid.

Potency—Pygeum extract can help those who suffer from BPH to improve sexual performance. BPH is often associated with erectile dysfunction and other sexual problems. In this case, pygeum can help men achieve full erections.

Saw Palmetto

Saw Palmetto is a small West Indian palm tree. It also grows in North America. The American Indians traditionally used Saw Palmetto berries as a tonic to support the body nutritionally, and was used by men as a fertility aid. Many herbalists consider it to be an aphrodisiac. This consideration may however be false.

Saw Palmetto has proven to be an effective supplement to help treat those who suffer from benign prostatic hyperplasia (BPH). Saw Palmetto inhibits the conversion of testosterone to DHT. It also inhibits DHT's activation through cellular binding. Moreover, recent studies show that Saw Palmetto possesses a strong anti-estrogenic effect. Estrogen accelerates prostate enlargement by inhibiting the elimination of DHT. However, according to these studies, Saw Palmetto possesses anti-androgenic activity, which means it may reduce the action of testosterone.

Saw Palmetto is still an open issue. While it seems to be an effective natural aid for prostate enlargement-related problems, it may, at the same time, reduce sex drive.

Conclusion:

Men who suffer from prostate enlargement-related problems should consider taking a combination of standardized Pygeum and standardized Saw Palmetto. In addition to alleviating BPH symptoms, a combination of these natural remedies helps to fight against estrogen and prolactin, reducing and eliminating their negative effects. When taken in early stages or before any symptoms occur, these natural aids may help prevent enlargement of the prostate and its related problems.

End Note:

If you suffer from prostate enlargement-related problems, you should seek professional medical help. You may also want to consider incorporating alternative healing methods in your treatment, such as the above herbal remedies, and making adjustments to your diet and lifestyle.

CHAPTER ELEVEN
Q & A

I'd like to address some frequently asked questions by those who have been practicing the Warrior Diet, and by others who are considering it.

Q: Does exercise influence when and how much you eat?

A: Yes it does. After exercising, particularly on an empty stomach, your insulin receptors are at peak sensitivity, your growth hormone is at the highest peak, and your glycogen reserves are depleted. This is the best time to eat. Your body is now ready to consume large amounts of food without gaining weight.

Q: What if you only exercise two days a week?

A: The Warrior Diet still works.

Q: Can you eat the same amount on the other five days as the two days you exercise? Maybe your body won't want as much.

A: You just asked and answered it. This is the only diet I know of that will eventually bring you to a natural rhythm, to feel your own cycle. In other words, you should crave and eat exactly what you need and as much as you need.

The days that you don't exercise, I truly believe that your hunger will be slightly less, and satiety will come more quickly. However, those who practice a whole day or two of undereating may need to eat more the following day, even if they didn't exercise.

Q: What about people who are unhealthy, or have a preexisting condition, such as hypoglycemia, where they're told they need to maintain their blood-sugar level, and so should eat throughout the day?

A: I have to say up-front that everyone, especially those who have preexisting conditions or are sick, should use common sense and consult with their physician before going on any diet. I presume that the majority of mainstream physicians will be opposed to the Warrior Diet, even for those who are healthy; regardless, I truly believe it will help most people, including those who suffer from hypoglycemia.

Q: What about children? Is this diet good for them?

A: The most important thing for children, in my opinion, is to make sure that they eat the right foods, which include raw vegetables, fruits, good-quality proteins, whole-grain carbohydrates, and good fats. Children need more fat then adults. Essential fatty acids are extremely important for babies and children's brain development and growth.

Children are like angels. Their natural instincts remain sharp if they're not corrupted. The problem, though, is that adults often try to crush their instincts. I believe that children have the Warrior Instinct, but many are forced to eat when they don't want to. As a general rule, when children are hungry they should eat, and when they aren't hungry, they shouldn't be forced to eat.

Children should not be on the Warrior Diet per se; however, having them eat fresh fruits and vegetables and drink freshly prepared juices made from veggies during the day would greatly benefit children.

Q: Most children are starving in the morning.

A: Remember, children are not on the Warrior Diet, so they should eat.

Q: Why do you think so many kids today only want to eat sweets, sugar-laden beverages, and fast food? And what can be done?

A: Many children develop aggressive tastes from a very early age. As a result, they're out of balance. When they're given or allowed to eat overly processed foods that contain too many additives with aggressive tastes, like sugar and other stimulators, or salt, or fried foods, etc., they begin to crave these unhealthy foods and become addicted to them. This is very destructive because these children lose their ability to enjoy the subtle tastes that come from nature. Not eating enough natural foods leads to deficiencies of essential nutrients. Chemicals in foods, such as petroleum-based pesticides, herbicides, nitrates, food colorings, and certain preservatives, as well as toxins, such as metal toxins (aluminum-based leavening) affect children much more than adults. Bad eating habits may lead to serious metabolic problems, retarded growth, and impaired mental development.

When children have unhealthy diets, I often recommend that parents try putting their kids on a moderated Warrior Diet, with a shorter period of undereating, where they're given raw fruits, veggies, and fresh juices made from them—and then feed them the right foods. Healthy instincts should eventually return and they'll begin to develop subtle tastes and enjoy healthy foods.

Q: What age is ideal for people to begin the Warrior Diet?

A: I think it's when they reach maturity. Until then, they should eat more frequent meals.

Q: At what age does one mature?

A: Sixteen to eighteen.

Q: So this diet is for people who are at least sixteen years old?

A: Yes. However, younger teens can practice a milder version of the Warrior Diet to experience the benefits of daily detoxification. As a guideline, maybe twice a week they could have fruit or fresh-fruit smoothies or freshly squeezed vegetable juices until lunchtime, and then have a meal. As mentioned earlier, Spartan boys were trained and fed like warriors, and they grew up to be strong, tough adults. This doesn't mean that I recommend a Spartan way of life. Nevertheless, this is an example that the Warrior Diet works for young adults.

Q: I've heard it said that vegetarians are more peaceful and spiritual then meat eaters. What do you think?

A: Some vegetarian-diet authors say that vegetarians are more peaceful than meat eaters, and that we'd live in a better world if people were vegetarian because they are also more spiritual than meat eaters. I strongly believe that this isn't so. Two of the bloodiest killers ever, Adolph Hitler and Joseph Stalin, were vegetarian. However, I can see where vegetarian advocates are coming from, and I respect their concerns about cruelty to animals and the environmental issue.

Q: How do you think people should deal with social and business events that involve meals while on the Warrior Diet?

A: While on the Warrior Diet, especially during the Undereating Phase, you'll feel alert and focused. This in itself is a big advantage for social and business-related events.

Here's my suggestion. For a breakfast meeting, stick to fresh fruit or a fresh fruit smoothie or juice, and coffee or tea. For a lunch meeting, veggie juices or the above are also appropriate. You can opt instead to have a salad with minimal dressing, and a small portion of protein, such as poached eggs, lean chicken breast, or fish. Dinnertime meals should be no problem. Just follow the overeating principles. People will be impressed with the amount of food you can eat during dinner without gaining fat. Explain that you're on the Warrior Diet. Many people today are on diets, so they should understand if you choose not to eat a typical breakfast or lunch. Don't feel a need to apologize. This is a free country.

Q: Can you have nuts or seeds during the Undereating Phase?

A: During the adaptation period, and days that you feel deprived, yes. Nuts and seeds are very good foods, particularly raw as opposed to roasted or seasoned. However, it's not ideal to eat them during the Undereating Phase because, although raw nuts and seeds won't activate your insulin, they may place pressure on your digestive system, and so not allow your body to completely detoxify.

Q: What about smoking and alcohol? Are they allowed?

A: The Warrior Diet is about diet, and it's also about a sense of freedom, from which many people feel deprived. When I say that this diet is a way of life, I mean that there are some profound ideas behind it that hopefully will improve your life as far as making priorities, defining goals, self-esteem, ambition, and creativity. I assume that those who follow the Warrior Diet have enough information to make the right choices, whether to drink alcohol or smoke, and if they choose to do either (or both) it's up to them. If you smoke or drink, the Warrior Diet will still help you to detoxify and stay in shape. The ability to make choices is what freedom is all about.

Q: People who drink a lot of alcohol are often overweight.

A: Alcohol-related problems, including stubborn fat, are discussed in Chapters 4 and 5.

Q: Do you have anything to say to those people who crave alcohol?

A: Being on the Warrior Diet may result in less alcohol consumption because the desire to drink to excess diminishes when you reach satiety from what you eat. I truly believe that excessive drinking has a lot to do with deprivation.

This said, having a glass or two of wine per day is usually fine for most people. As mentioned before, great warriors in the past used to drink wine every night.

Q: Jews and Muslims fast once a year. How does this relate to the Warrior Diet?

A: People in the past were aware that if they wanted to cleanse and reach a spiritual state of mind, fasting was the route to take. For Muslims, Ramadan means fasting during the day and eating at night. In my opinion, Ramadan is an example of an old, traditional fast that is similar to the Warrior Diet. People who fast during Ramadan say that they feel physically, mentally, and spiritually rejuvenated. Fasting for Jews, such as on Yom Kippur, is meant to be a spiritual cleansing; getting away from the materialistic world is a way to cleanse one's body and spirit.

Q: What should I do with all this new energy that I have?

A: If you do suffer—and I say again "suffer"—from too much energy, then go and find yourself a life. It's best that I stick to the subject of diet and not become a preacher. I truly believe that once the Warrior Instinct is triggered, people gain more courage to try things they may have been afraid to attempt before. They become more adventurous, more romantic, more creative, and more competitive. So the question about what to do with all this extra energy is, in my opinion, irrelevant. If you ask a champion athlete "What do you do with your extra energy that comes from all this training?" they'll likely tell you, "Get out o' here."

Q: What about those who find it hard to calm down or sleep at night?

A: If you find it difficult to calm down at night, you may not be consuming enough carbohydrates.

Enzymes and Live-Food Enzymes

Q: Who needs enzymes?

A: Everybody needs enzymes. Young people have a higher enzyme pool in their bodies than older people. The older we get, the less enzymes we have, so enzyme supplementation is often needed.

Q: When is the best time to take enzymes?

A: I always suggest taking enzymes on an empty stomach or just before a meal because this gives them time to reload your system and reach your blood. As I've mentioned before, according to research studies, enzymes (such as protease enzymes) effectively reduce inflammation and may also have the ability to destroy pathogenic bacteria, viruses, sick cells, and tumors, so they may have a healing, anticancerous effect.

Q: How many should I take?

A: It depends on the product's manufacturer. Check the label and experiment. One-to-four capsules before your meal is usually sufficient. Monitor yourself for what works best. You may try to increase the dosage gradually. For some people, high dosage works better.

Q: What are the best enzymes to take?

A: The enzymes that have the most healing effects are protease enzymes (enzymes that break down protein, thereby aiding in the purification of the blood and the intestinal tract). For example, bromelein (derived from pineapple) is a protease enzyme. In addition to breaking down protein, it's helpful for reducing water retention, inflammation, and therefore helpful in the healing process. Bromelein works like an antioxidant. All protease enzymes, including papaine (derived from papayas) and tripzine (pancreatic protease) have an antioxidant effect. It's preferable to take a combination of protease enzymes rather than just one, but they will still be effective in both cases. Some people believe, including myself, that plant enzymes are the most effective because they contain the widest variety. Although plant enzymes do contain proteolic enzymes, unfortunately they're not high in them. But the variety of enzymes in plant enzymes is enormous, so they are wonderful for you nonetheless. Moreover, plant enzymes are more stable in high temperature or highly acidic environments.

Q: Are live food enzymes good enough?

A: If you want to ensure maximum potency, especially since people today consume so much processed food, I think it's best to consume live foods and take digestive enzyme supplements, as well as probiotics.

> **Warrior-zyme** is a potent combination of vital live enzymes. It's high in undenatured protease and lipase, essential for detoxification, digestion, and proper metabolism. For more on this, go to the "Warrior Diet Nutritional Supplements."

Q: Are there other enzymes?

A: Yes, there are antioxidant enzymes. The most important ones are SOD (Super Oxide Dismutase) and reduced glutathione, both of which the body produces naturally.

• SOD (Super Oxide Dismutase):

In order to produce enough SOD, your body needs the minerals zinc, manganese, and copper, as well as probiotics (beneficial bacteria). Besides being a super antioxidant and a first defense against free radicals, SOD is also vital for your potency and ability to become sexually aroused. Healthy cells contain SOD, which protects them from nitric oxide (NO—a natural substance that the body produces. Nitric oxide is necessary for regulating your blood pressure, and is vital for your brain and heart. Moreover, without it men cannot produce an erection or be potent. Nitric oxide is believed to have an anticancerous effect, because when it reaches cancer cells, it may destroy them. In other words, without nitric oxide you're dead, and without SOD, this nitric oxide mechanism doesn't work.

• Glutathione:

Glutathione is another vital antioxidant enzyme the body produces. The glutathione pool in your body is an index determining how healthy you are. Your body should produce glutathione naturally from precursors if you eat the right amount of foods containing cysteine, glycine, and glutamine.

Unfortunately, cysteine is such a sensitive protein that most processing destroys it. Foods such as bean sprouts, cruciferous vegetables, and minimally processed dairy, all contain cysteine. Egg yolks are another good natural source of cysteine. Whey and colostrum should be too. Maintaining a high pool of cysteine in your body is a good example of why it's so important to keep food live and potent.

Glutathione supplements are available, but your body should be able to produce it naturally by nourishing it with the right foods. Certain sea plants like spirulina and chlorella, as well as raw meat and raw fish, do contain glutathione, but it's usually destroyed by digestive enzymes in the stomach. Therefore the best way to keep glutathione levels high is by ingesting the right natural precursors so your body will be able to produce it by itself.

Glycine and glutamine appear in all complete protein foods, such as animal meats, and dairy.

Chapter Twelve
The Warrior
Workout

Exercising is essential for maximizing the Warrior Diet's effects—it's the bridge between the two main phases, undereating and overeating.

Have you ever asked yourself...

- **What is my physical potential?**
- **Have I tried to reach my limits?**
- **Do I feel strong in certain areas, but weak in others?**
- **Am I quick enough?**
- **Can I jump high a few times without falling apart?**
- **Can I sprint for more than 30 seconds without collapsing?**
- **Do I know the difference between being *strong* and being *tough*?**
- **Do I like what I see in the mirror?**

The goal of this training program is to enable you to reach your body's potential, and maintain it. What I call *"body potential" is based on function— not fashion.* The emphasis will be to activate and strengthen the most essential and functional muscle groups. In the past, warriors were aware of the importance of a functional body, and its effect on balance, speed, explosive moves, strength, and endurance. Sport training in ancient Greece and Rome was based on exercises that mimicked warfare or hunting activities.

The modern concept of *training to failure* (training until reaching complete muscle exhaustion) was definitely not a warrior way. Failure was simply not allowed. As mentioned in the "Lessons from History" chapter, Romans, Spartans, and Greeks were lean and muscular. Being lean was a must. Building a lean muscular body was a result of functional strength training.

To accelerate strength and speed without adding unnecessary bulk, a special exercise routine is needed. The Warrior Workout addresses this. It works on body-balance, joints, and stabilizing muscles, and on the ability to adapt to controlled fatigue (the ability to control your fatigue while training, and not letting fatigue control you). This exercise routine closely mimics the daily activities of ancient warriors.

The Warrior Workout deserves a book to itself, but since there's not enough space, I'll focus on the foundation, the most important elements, and the basics. The information provided is sufficient to get you started and on your way.

This exercise program is based on cycling between intense resistance and high velocity (explosive moves and speed). It includes special supersets to maximize the natural synergistic effect of different muscle groups. This routine incorporates both aerobic and resistance training, and is designed for those who have no time to waste.

Part One of this chapter covers the principles of the workout. At the end of Part One, I include preworkout and recovery meals. Part Two focuses on specific exercises, designed to help you follow the workout principles.

Lean 'n' Mean for a Lifetime

A few years ago I was watching a TV interview with former Olympic champions. The program showed clips of these athletes during the peak of their careers, and the contrast in how they looked then and now startled me; it was really surprising to see how out of shape most of them had become. For instance, the ex-Olympic champion sprinter Vladimir Borosov, the fastest man in the world during the 1970s, was lean and well defined. Now a businessman, he has a big belly, and looks heavy and sluggish.

It got me thinking how competitive athletes in many sports, such as football, soccer, boxing, and swimming, who were also "lean 'n' mean" during their competitive careers, often look completely out of shape years later. This "syndrome" is also found among ex-combat soldiers. While serving, they're in great shape, but when no longer engaged in a daily training routine, they often gain weight, and look softer.

Why does this happen so frequently? In my opinion, athletes and soldiers, who lose their drive to stay in shape, tend to do so because their minds and bodies simply became overexhausted and depleted from years of training.

Exercising, training, and any other physical activity for that matter, whether competitive, combative, or not, should be thought of in a larger context—what works for you over the course of your life. A progressive training routine will only be successful if you can live with it; it should energize you and help trigger your "Warrior Instinct," with the drive to continually improve yourself. Without this, sooner or later you'll burn out.

The Warrior Workout Goals

- *Build a functional, lean, muscular body*
- *Accelerate your metabolism*
- *Burn fat*
- *Develop strength, speed, and endurance*
- *Improve your body image*
- *Improve your balance*
- *Improve your posture*
- *Sharpen your instincts*
- *Accelerate your alertness and drive (competitive aggression)*

The Warrior Workout Principles

1. *Make strength-training priorities: joints and back*
2. *Cycle between intense resistance and high velocity (explosive moves)*
3. *Train under "controlled fatigue"*
4. *Do not train to reach complete muscle failure*
5. *Make your workout short*

Part One

Principle #1: Make strength-training priorities: joints and back.

The first step of a progressive exercise routine is to make priorities. It's necessary to understand the priorities, especially if your goal is to gain strength rather than size or bulk.

Roman, Spartan, Macedonian, and Greek warriors were lean and light, yet their performance during war campaigns required a great deal of power and strength. A Roman soldier typically carried 40–60 lbs. of arms and equipment on his back while marching thirty or forty miles a day. He moved through tough geographical terrain that forced him to climb up and down hills, march in water, and run through rocky fields. Sometimes after a long march, this Roman warrior had to fight for hours, and then set up camp. What made these lean and light people so physically strong? I believe it was due to their joint and back strength.

Back Strength (for carrying weapons)

For an ancient warrior, back strength was essential. During the Olympian games, which go as far back as the sixth century B.C., Greek athletes competed with full body armor, including helmets, shields, and javelins. Running while fully armed requires back strength. This method of training is still popular among Marines and other combat units today.

Joint Strength (jumping, swinging, stabbing, slashing, pushing, pulling)

Fighting activities such as jumping, fencing, stabbing, slashing, and swinging are all related to joint and tendon strength. Tendons and ligaments connect the muscles to the bones. Weak tendons compromise muscle elasticity. Joint strength depends on the strength of essential muscle groups and tissues, which are responsible for all joint movements. strength of essential muscle groups and tissues, which are responsible for all joint movements.

The top priorities, then, for a functional lean body should be strengthening your shoulders, wrists, elbows, waist, abdominals, buttocks, knees, ankles, and back.

Shoulder strength was necessary for slashing and stabbing. A Macedonian and Roman phalanx infantryman was supposed to be able to stop a horse attack with his shield. Push (press) and pull activities needed shoulder, elbow, and back strength. Swings required waist, back, and knee strength. Running or jumping while carrying a heavy load needed back, knee, buttock, and ankle strength. Fighting with a sword required a strong grip—which meant strong wrists and forearms.

In short, making priorities is essential for a complete Warrior Workout. To develop a lean and functional body, back and joint strength should be your top priorities. Basic training exercises that specialize in back and joint strength are covered in Part Two of this chapter.

> It doesn't matter how big your muscles are if your tendons are weak; you won't be able to reach your peak level of strength. Moreover, having an overgrown muscle belly, combined with weak tendons may lead to severe injuries, such as torn muscles.

Principle #2: Cycle between intense resistance (strength) and high velocity (explosive moves).

During army campaigns, soldiers were under intense physical strain. Ancient warriors always had to be ready for a fight. Fighting face-to-face often required the ability to push and pull strongly, as well as master explosive stabbing or slashing movements.

Roman and Macedonian infantrymen used the shield as a pushing board against their enemy. A typical combat strategy was to push an opponent so hard that he'd lose his balance, and at the same time deliver a quick explosive hit with a sword (slash or stab) that was meant to wound or kill. Intense pulling skills were needed for wrestling when warriors fought holding one another. A strong pull over the opponent's neck could throw him down, or pull him into a dagger. In other words, both power moves and explosive moves were necessary for an ancient warrior engaged in combat activities.

This training routine isn't meant to prepare you for a fight, though it might very well be helpful for martial artists. The routine's purpose is to mimic the basic functions of a warrior body—to be strong and quick.

The second principle of this workout is to cycle between intense resistance (strength) and high velocity (explosive moves). By following this exercise routine, you'll be able to train your mind to adapt to intense resistance through special heavyweight training cycles, and to react quickly with explosive exercises such as cleans, frog jumps, high jumps, kicks, and sprints.

Controlled Intense Resistance

To gain strength, you have to lift heavy weights. I consider a heavy weight to be a load that you can lift for no more than 5–6 reps. Heavy weight is a relative matter. For a beginner, a heavy load could be 20 lbs. For a trained person, it might be 200 lbs. Choose whatever is appropriate for you.

Lifting light weights won't lead to anything other than burning calories; however, there are some exceptions to this statement, such as leg workouts—when a heavy weight may compromise the right form. I'll explain this further in Part Two.

Gaining strength is a matter of adaptation, perseverance, and skill. The goal here is to give your brain a signal that a heavy weight—with high tension—must be handled. Once your brain adapts to a certain degree of physical tension, it's a sign that you've gained some strength and will be able to gradually increase the weight load.

Strength is the ability to handle tension in time and space.

The factors that determine strength are:

1. Tension – The weight (intensity)
2. Time – The time under tension (volume)
3. Space – The length of the motion (form)

You must follow these three parameters to maximize your strength gain. The training program in Part Two is designed to give you basic exercise routines that activate all three factors: intensity, form, and volume. To gain strength, you need to alternate the weight loads and number of sets per session. Keeping the right form is also a must. Since heavy sets are low reps, the way to build volume is to incorporate a few heavy sets with a short rest in between (or no rest), which builds into a giant intense superset.

This training routine is built on body function, not on body parts. It incorporates different muscle groups, such as antagonistic muscles, while maximizing the synergetic effect of body movements (such as pushes and pulls). As stated, don't waste your time with light weights—or you might as well do something more useful instead, like washing dishes or gardening. If you want to train like a warrior, go heavy, but do it wisely.

I call this workout method "controlled resistance" because it will enable you to control the intensity and volume of the exercises and, therefore, you'll gradually improve.

High Velocity (Explosive Moves)

Explosive moves are not an integral part of a typical bodybuilding routine. Just go to any neighborhood gym and watch how people train. Very few, if any, try explosive moves such as clean and press or clean jerks. High jumps, frog jumps, or one-leg jumps are explosive training methods, which don't hold muster for an average Joe who's trying to pump his thighs by doing heavy squats half the way.

In my opinion, explosive strength is essential for a lean and functional body. Ballistic exercises, like clean and press, work your whole body. They require explosive strength, balance, and skill. Following a training program that incorporates different explosive exercises, with a gradual increase of weight and volume, will tone your body, making it stronger and more agile. There are quite a few variations for high-velocity training. I'll cover the most basic exercises, which I believe will stimulate your mind and body to adapt to high-velocity exercises, and gain real functional and instinctual strength.

High-velocity exercises (which often include power lifting) are very demanding. They involve your mind, body, and your instincts. This kind of training should be done once a week. If you've already tried it, you know how it feels to do a few repetitive heavy sets of, say, clean presses. It takes all you have. But whatever you put in, you're sure to get back. For me, high-velocity training days are fun. When I do them I feel like I'm playing with power.

Power and strength are what really counted for a warrior. Size was not an issue. Thousands of years ago, wrestlers and boxers disregarded the body-weight factor when they fought in the Games. That, in my opinion, mimicked real-life situations. This training program won't teach you the fighting skills needed to face a giant opponent. But it definitely will help you face yourself in the mirror.

Principle # 3: Train Under Controlled Fatigue (train to be tough)

Controlled fatigue is a warrior-training concept. Being able to function properly when fatigued was critical to warrior life. Romans believed the winner of a fight was the one who could endure the most pain. As discussed in "Lessons from History," Roman warriors inflicted pain and torture on themselves in order to prepare for the real thing. During war, an ancient warrior, especially an infantryman, had to endure constant intense physical pain and mental stress. War campaigns typically forced a soldier to perform combat activities under prolonged fatigue.

Army training is not the same as sport training. The goals of sport training are to make athletes stronger and quicker. Conversely, the goal of army training is to first and foremost make soldiers tougher. Being tough requires the ability to endure stress, whether physical or mental, for a prolonged time.

Sometimes, training to be tough may come at the expense of gaining strength, at least in the short run. However, in the long run, what I call controlled-fatigue training pays back generously. A body trained under controlled fatigue learns how to adapt to long periods of intense pressure without reaching failure. It's this intense, long, pressure with the "fatigue factor" that forces your body to make physical and mental priorities. To say it differently, under controlled fatigue, there's "no time or place for bullshit." A man really learns about himself when faced with such conditions.

When faced with constant intense strain, your body will instinctively do only the most important functional moves, which will deliver maximum strength. Fancy moves are useless when your body's instincts kick in.

When the going gets tough, the tough get going

The more you train under controlled fatigue, the more you can handle stress. As I've said, this is a key factor in what makes a person tough. Controlled-fatigue training programs incorporate pre-exhausting exercises or aerobic activities, followed by intense resistance training. It also incorporates giant supersets built on short, intense, heavy sets. All the above can be cycled with different volumes (length of supersets) and levels of intensity (amount of weight lifted). Controlled-fatigue training can be done one day a week, or three- to- five days per week.

If your goal is to get tougher, then let the going get tough. In my opinion, you may be able to gain much strength when alternating between controlled-fatigue and strength-training days. For example, one week of controlled-fatigue training followed by one week of pure strength training will enable you to strengthen muscle groups while stimulating neuromuscular units not fully activated prior to this routine. Eventually, it all leads to a win-win situation, because you'll become tougher, stronger, and, most importantly, more in tune with your own instincts. If you've reached a plateau in your current workout regime, this is one way to break it. Controlled-fatigue training, if nothing else, will accelerate your mind-body connection in an instinctual way, enabling you to react and perform at any time.

A relatively long time under pressure doesn't make the workout long.

Controlled-fatigue training isn't necessarily a long workout routine. It puts your body under intense tension, which lasts for up to a few minutes. When a typical 10-rep set takes 30 seconds, a giant superset under controlled fatigue could take 3-to-5 minutes, and maybe even more. A relatively long time under intense pressure doesn't make the workout session long. Quite the opposite. As you'll see in Principle # 5, the workout should be short. You should be able to finish resistance training after 20–30 minutes.

Lactic-Acid Efficiency

As a last note, I'd like to briefly cover the effect of this routine on lactic-acid efficiency. Under controlled-fatigue training, your body becomes more and more efficient in metabolizing lactic acid into energy. The burn that you feel in your muscles when working out is a result of accumulating lactic acid in your muscles. Lactic acid is a byproduct of glucose metabolism. Under prolonged intense exercise, too much of this substance may block your muscles' ability to contract. This is the bad news.

The good news is that lactic acid converts into pyruvate, which, according to recent research, boosts energy and accelerates metabolism. Moreover, by decreasing the pH in your tissues, lactic acid could be a major factor in boosting your anabolic hormones. A physically trained person's body should be more efficient in metabolizing lactic acid into energy and, therefore, able to handle longer periods of intense exercise and recuperate faster than an untrained body. Controlled-fatigue training is one of the best and most efficient methods to boost your metabolism and burn fat. For those interested in accelerating the Warrior Diet's effects, this is the way to do it.

Principle #4: Do not train to reach failure

As stated, training to reach failure is not a warrior way. For a warrior, failure was not allowed. Ancient warriors, especially Spartans and Romans, considered failure worse than death. A Roman soldier was ready at any time to fight until the end. Surrendering was a disgrace.

The concept of not reaching failure has much more to do with your mental state than your physical state. When you train your body to avoid failure, you'll learn by trial and error how to keep moving and improving, without losing control. Conversely, when you chronically train to reach failure, your mind will surrender every time it feels that your body has reached its limit. Subconsciously, your mind will "prefail" before your body, because that's the way it was trained. When you're used to failure, it stops your body from crossing barriers. In other words, if you train to reach failure, you will fail.

Training not to reach failure does not necessarily mean you won't fail. It does mean training in a way that encourages you to avoid failure — by stopping one step before reaching this dead end. While training, you may continually encounter a point where your body can no longer perform. This is a way to study your current limits, so next time you'll know when to stop. Stopping one rep before failure gives your brain the signal that you're still in full control.

Failure brings its own psychosomatic effects. Muscle failure during training is often a result of a defense mechanism. Your brain gives your muscles an order to fail, out of fear of injury. The reason why ancient warriors tortured themselves was mainly to conquer the fear of pain. Conquering the fear of pain or injury could be the main reason why a 130 lb. Olympian weightlifter could successfully press 300 lb. weights above his head. Training to failure remains popular among many bodybuilders and athletes today. This issue is controversial, especially for those who are mainly interested in gaining strength.

Those who believe in reaching failure argue that only by pushing to the limit—meaning reaching failure—will you be able to gain muscle size. According to this line of thinking, it's the last two failed reps that count. Training to reach failure needs spotting, by a trainer or a training partner. Without spotting, it's almost impossible to exercise the effect of the last two failed reps. I'm not trying to dismiss this method of training, because it might work well as far as gaining muscle size. However, I do question it as far as strength is concerned.

My points are simple:

1. When you depend on a spotter to lift you up every time that you reach failure, then you fail to reach your own limits.

2. By chronically reaching failure, you exhaust yourself, and therefore rob yourself of your physical strength potential and mental aggression to go on.

A good workout session should charge your energy, not deplete it. Knowing you will not reach failure is a state of mind. This state of mind should be yours before, during, and especially after, your workout. You should at all times feel you can "kick ass."

Principle #5: Make your workout short.

Make your workout short and intense. Long resistance-workout sessions may compromise your strength and hormonal levels. There's enough research that shows how after 45 minutes of intense, resistance training, there is a decline in blood testosterone. You should finish your workout while your hormones are at a peak level. Manipulating your hormones is one of the Warrior Diet goals, and it should be the same goal for the Warrior Workout.

The timeframe for constructive intense resistance training is between 20–45 minutes. The Warrior Workout is designed to be no longer than 20–30 minutes per session of resistance training.

Short resistance-training sessions are more practical, and for busy people this is a great advantage. To be successful, a progressive workout program should be easy to follow—one you can live with on a daily basis. If you know why you're training and how to do it, you're almost there. Knowing that it'll only take 20-45 minutes — and then you can go back to the locker room— is encouraging. Short sessions make it easier to monitor and stay focused. When you finish each workout you should be able to say, as Julius Caesar once declared: "Veni, vidi, vici" —"I came, I saw, I conquered."

Aerobics

Aerobic training is an essential part of the Warrior Workout. The goals of aerobics are to:

- *Improve endurance and speed*
- *Accelerate fat-burning*
- *Prefatigue the body for controlled-fatigue training*

Aerobics can be cycled between short sessions of intense intervals, such as sprints, that last for 10–15 minutes, and longer endurance fat-burning sessions lasting 20–45 minutes. Doing aerobics on an empty stomach will accelerate the Warrior Diet effects of boosting your growth hormone, depleting your glycogen reserves, and accelerating fat burning.

Aerobics exercises are covered in Part Two of this chapter.

Preworkout and Recovery Meals

Preworkout and recovery meals are optional. The logic behind these meals is to minimize the catabolic and stress effects of the workout, replenish muscles, and accelerate the anabolic effects after the workout.

Always make sure you drink plenty of water before, during, and immediately after your workout.

Preworkout meals are best for those people interested in gaining muscle size.

Preworkout Meal Principle:

To supply the body with nutrients which will minimize the catabolic and stress effects of the workout, without boosting insulin.

Preworkout Goals:
- *Minimize Catabolism*
- *Reduce Stress*
- *Boost Neurotransmitters (Alertness)*
- *Keep Hormones at a Peak Level*
- *Keep Insulin Low*

Preworkout Meal
Warrior Growth Serum

Warrior Growth Serum is a proprietary blend of low-temperature, air-dried, undenatured organic colostrum protein with other essential nutrients. Warrior Growth Serum is specially designed to accelerate growth and immunity. More on Warrior Growth Serum can be found in the "Warrior Nutritional Supplements" chapter.

I generally recommend taking 5–20g of Warrior Growth Serum before your workout. This powder tastes so good in its natural state that I scoop out the desired amount with a spoon and eat it plain. If you choose to chew the powder, the stickiness will dissolve in your mouth in a minute. You can also mix Warrior Growth Serum with some water. It's up to you. For those interested in muscle growth, boosting immunity, and fat loss, this is the best choice.

Preworkout Meal Alternatives

Those who skip a preworkout meal can have coffee or tea instead. Good, fresh coffee is a wonderful natural stimulator before a workout. Caffeine, which is a strong alkaloid, can boost your metabolism up to 20 percent higher, and therefore further accelerate the fat-burning effects. Caffeine boosts dopamine (a major brain neurotransmitter, giving you a feeling of alertness and well-being). In general, a shot or two of good espresso will do it; or a cup of, say, English Breakfast.

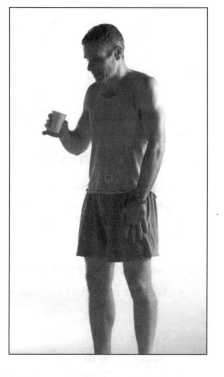

Caffeine works best when ingested on an empty stomach, with no carbs. In my opinion, adding one teaspoon of unrefined sugar won't change much for active people, but to be on the safe side, skip the carbs if you can. Sugar may fluctuate your insulin and as a result may cause a hypoglycemic reaction during the workout, causing you to feel dizzy, drained, or exhausted. You can add milk, preferably milk foam, to the coffee or tea. Too much milk will slow the absorption of the caffeine and may cause an upset stomach during the workout.

Those sensitive to coffee can also substitute it with guarana. Guarana tea is a natural source of pure caffeine without the acidity. It's a mild pickup. I find guarana to be too alkaline, so I mix it with ginger. Guarana with ginger tastes better to me. Guarana is sold in many health-food stores.

Exercising on an Empty Stomach— The Fat-Burning Factor

If gaining muscle mass is not your goal, then the preworkout meal isn't necessary. Training on an empty stomach will accelerate the undereating effects of the diet. As discussed in previous chapters, when you exercise during a controlled fast, your body's main source of energy will come from burning fat. People who suffer from stubborn fat should take advantage of the "exercise on empty" factor. This accelerates fat burning in areas such as under the skin, which diet alone won't accomplish as rapidly. For those interested in having lean definition, this is the best way to go.

Recovery Meals

Recovery meals are more important than preworkout meals. After your workout, your hormones are at a peak level and your insulin is stabilized. This is the best time to eat.

Recovery Meal Principle:
- *To accelerate the anabolic effects of the workout.*

Recovery Meal Goals:
- *Accelerate growth*
- *Replenish nutrients to depleted muscles*
- *Boost immunity*

Recovery Meals:

I highly recommend taking a mineral supplement before and right after your workout to avoid mineral deficiency-related symptoms and to alkalize the body. Exercise acidifies the body. Over-acidity may deactivate the effects of growth hormones on your body.

Warrior Milk (protein meal)

Warrior Milk is a proprietary blend of undenatured, specially processed whey protein with growth serum. Warrior Milk may be the best alternative to other commercial over-processed protein powders. This warrior protein meal will supply your body with the nutrients and proteins essential for growth and recuperation. More on Warrior Milk is found in the "Warrior Nutritional Supplements" chapter.

I generally recommend having one serving of Warrior Milk immediately after your workout. I keep it in the locker room. This protein meal contains a natural sweetener to enhance flavor and accelerate the absorption of nutrients to your starving muscles. It tastes delicious whether you choose to chew the powder on its own, or mix it with water.

Warrior Growth Serum

Warrior Growth Serum is good both as a preworkout meal, and as a recovery meal. This protein meal is highly concentrated with growth factors and immune factors that naturally support the metabolic and anabolic process before and after your workout. See "Preworkout Meals" for more on this. I generally recommend one serving before and after your workout.

The best time to have a recovery meal is right after the workout. Then, about an hour later — or whenever you start feeling hungry — go for your evening meal. If you workout in the morning or during the day, it's usually best to have a recovery meal right after the workout and then continue to follow the Undereating Phase until evening. This should sustain you for the rest of the day, without compromising the goals of the Undereating Phase. However, people who feel the need for whole protein foods during the day can have eggs (preferably poached), fish, or lean cuts of meat.

Part Two
The Workout

Proper breathing is critical for performance and overall health. Breathing deeply alkalizes your system, and therefore reduces the acid-stress factor on your body. Deep inhalations followed by deep exhalations supply your tissues with vital oxygen, while eliminating carbon dioxide. Conversely, shallow or improper breathing causes an oxygen deficiency and retention of carbon dioxide, which accelerates the build-up of carbonic acid in the blood. Poor oxygenation to the cells, and an overly acidic system, leads to muscle fatigue and stiffness, and stress-related exhaustion.

Abdominals

Abdominal muscles (abs) are divided into three main muscle groups:

1. Rectus Abdominus (the six pack)

2. Serratus Anterior (sides of the upper abs)

3. External Obliques (sides of the lower abs)

However, all abdominal muscles are bound together by connective tissues into one large muscle.

Abdominal training is a controversial issue. There are differing opinions about abdominal muscle development. Trainers who use specific ab-training methods often try to prove that theirs are superior to other ab routines. People who want to define their midsection spend much time on ab-training methods such as sit-ups, crunches, reverse crunches, hanging leg raises, Roman chair sit-ups, ab-flexor machines, rollers, and more.

The problem with many of these methods is not the efficiency of the exercises, but the fact that they're built on isolating one ab part or another. Isolating one part of a large muscle group may cause imbalance and weakness in other parts of the same muscle. That's why it's so important to understand that abs are, in fact, one large muscle group working as a unit. They have primary functions, essential for body movements and posture. Let me put it simply: the prime function of the abdominals is to stabilize the midsection of your body, and thus protect your organs and support your spine. Abs should always be toned and ready for action. Sluggish, soft abs will cause vulnerability and dysfunction.

As a stabilizer of your midsection, the ab muscles are responsible for all waist movements such as swings, twists, bends, or crunches. The stabilizing function of abs manifests itself clearly when you're engaged in explosive moves such as punching or kicking. Notice that without the reflexive tightening of your abs, you can't deliver a powerful punch or an explosive kick. Abdominal muscles respond instinctively to explosive or powerful frontal arm and leg movements. By contracting, and thus stabilizing, your midsection as a solid column or basis for all explosive moves, ab muscles protect your spine from the rebound forces of your arm and leg movements. To perform with maximum strength, you need to tighten your midsection. A soft or weak waist may force you to compromise on your ability to lift weights, kick, or punch. Moreover, without abdominal support, you wouldn't be able to stand or walk.

We tend to take ab function for granted. A trained gymnast will tell you that there's no way to successfully stand on your hands without tightening your midsection. If your abs and lower back are loose, your body will collapse. This fact is not just true for standing on your hands. Without abdominal support, as stated above, you wouldn't be able to sing, "I'm still standing." Martial artists and boxers are particularly aware of this.

A trained warrior is ready at any time to absorb a hit on his midsection. A warrior's abs instinctively contract to protect the spine and inside organs, while absorbing the punch or kick. Habitual reflexive toning of the ab muscles enables a warrior to instinctively swing, punch, or kick whenever necessary.

The Warrior Posture

A trained warrior often adapts a unique posture, which I call the "Warrior Posture." People engaged in intense physical activities, like martial artists, gymnasts, some professional competitive

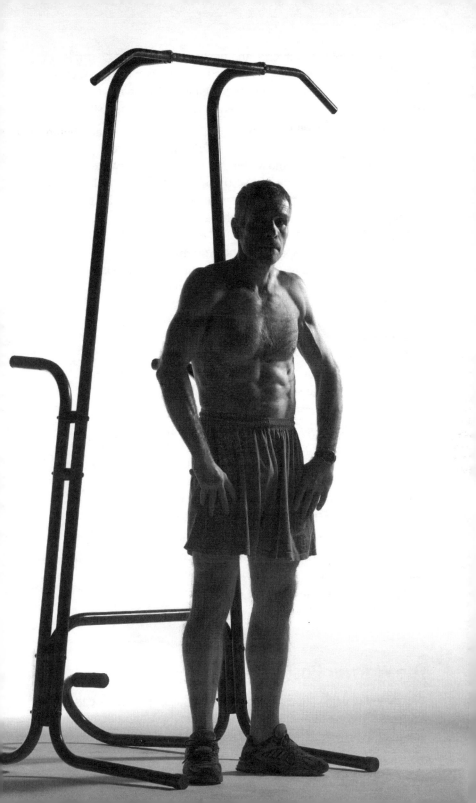

athletes, oreven hard laborers for that matter often obtain a posture where their abs are slightly flexed, and their back is ever so slightly bent forward. This isn't a fashion model or dandy posture; it looks quite different. Some fashion models, as well as many guys who want to look tall, often push their chest out, pumping air into their rib cage, and try to walk as high as they can. This stiff walk, without a bounce, makes them more vulnerable. When I see people walk this way (usually men), particularly if they have a belly, it often reminds me of a strolling penguin.

What I call a "Warrior Posture" has nothing to do with posing in front of a mirror. It is, in fact, the result of a natural adaptation of the body to tough, physical strain. I'm not trying to persuade people to walk like warriors. I'm just trying to point out what a "Warrior Posture" is and how it's naturally designed to enhance agility. If you find yourself instinctively walking like a warrior, I'd say it's a clear sign that you've been around the block a few times. You're always at heightened alertness, and are ready for action at all times.

Okay, enough of all this bravado. Let's go to the exercises.

Ab Exercises: 1 Set

There are many variations of abdominal training. I cover the basic ones—definitely enough to get you started. Let me note here that basic doesn't mean easy. The Warrior Abs Routine activates all abdominal muscles in one giant superset and is, in fact, quite intense. It works on the serratus anterior muscles, the external obliques, the upper and lower rectus abdominis, and the connective tissues between the serratus, the obliques, and the rectus abdominus.

I think of this giant superset as a double cheeseburger. The bun is hanging leg-raise exercises. The double cheeseburger is crunch and reverse crunch exercises. It takes about 2–3 minutes, and everything that you have to finish a set. All you need is one set per day, on each workout day. As noted, the main function of the abs is to stabilize the midsection while protecting the spine and inside organs. Therefore, it's important to incorporate isometric exercises together with isotonic exercises.

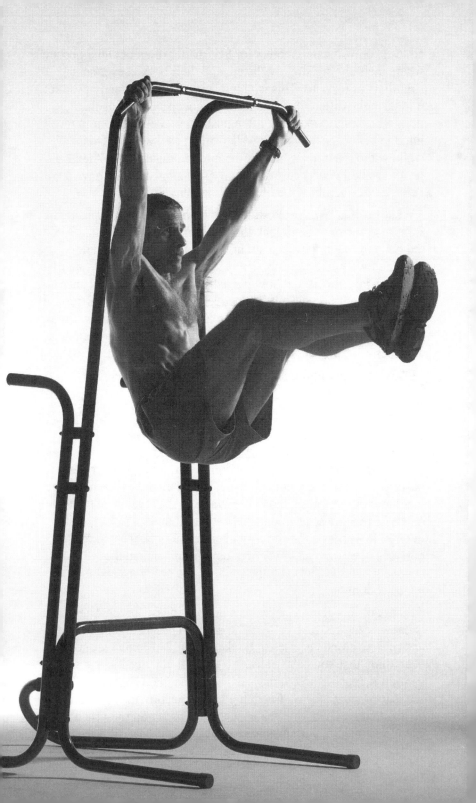

- *Isometric*—static exercises that contract the muscles without shortening them.

- *Isotonic*—dynamic exercises that involve movement, and shortening (thickening) of the muscles.

Most people are weak in the side layers of the abs (the serratus and the external obliques). In addition to the aesthetic factor (these muscles give you fine definition, and a compact look), the serratus and the obliques are necessary for all swings, punches, kicks and leg raises. Having tight, strong sides will give you a flat and strong midsection. I believe that the best way to work the sides of your midsection is by incorporating special isometric (freezing) exercises with isotonic exercises (movement). Static intense pressure on the abs will trigger a reflex of maximum contraction, thus forcing them to function the way they're meant to—as stabilizers and protectors of your midsection.

Ab Superset: 1 Set—Hanging Leg Raise

Stand under a chin-up bar. Grab the bar with both hands, palms down, at about shoulder width. Hang. Your feet should be flexed, pointing forward. Slowly raise your feet toward your hands. Your toes should touch the bar. Advanced exercisers should try to keep their legs almost straight. Beginners can bend their legs to ease the tension.

Slowly lower your legs to eye-level. Keep your legs at that level for 10 seconds while rotating them with small movements: 2-3 to the right side and 2-3 to the left side. Slowly lower your legs to about a 45-degree angle with your torso and then lift them up again to eye level. Try to keep them at about eye-level for another 5-10 seconds. If it's too hard, bend your knees. Slowly bring your legs down to 45 degrees. Bend your knees and then bring them up to your chest, keep them for 3 seconds and then bring them down. Repeat 5-10 times. When done, bring them up to your chest again. Keep your knees as high and as close to your chest as you can,

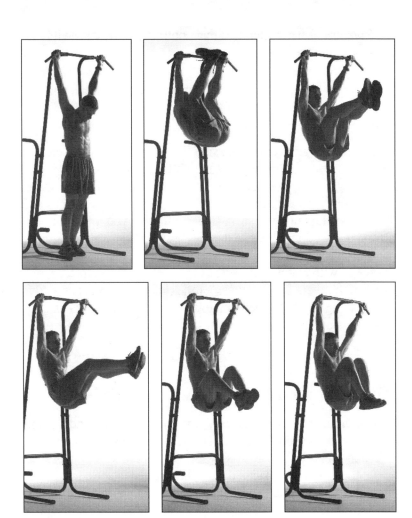

and keep them at that position for another 5-10 seconds. When you're done, you'll feel your lower abs and sides burning.

If you haven't collapsed by now, bring your legs down slowly. Now, grab a bench. You're going to do the crunches as part of this exercise; no resting in between.

Crunches: 10 reps

Sit on a bench with your knees just above the edge of the bench. Your feet should be flat on the floor. Lie down on your

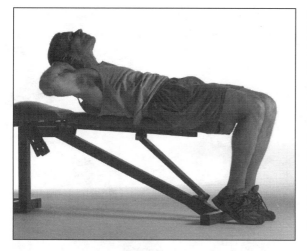

back and hams. Your hands should be behind your head, and your elbows should point to the side. Slowly lift your torso as high as you can.

Don't bounce, or use any momentum. Use your abs only. When you reach the top, stay for 5-7 seconds, and on each second count, try to squeeze the crunch as if trying to reach with your chin farther and farther forward. Your chin should be raised slightly and your elbows pointing to the sides at all times. Go slowly down to starting position without losing muscle contraction. Always keep your abs contracted. Repeat 10 times.

When you're done, start reverse crunches; no resting in between sets.

Reverse Crunches:
5-7 reps and partial reps

Grab the bench with your hands a few inches behind your head. Slowly bring your knees up above your head. Push through your rib cage at all times. Don't jerk or use momentum, but always keep your knees bent during this exercise. When you reach the top, slowly lower your legs. If you have advanced training, try to lower your legs while they're fully extended (fully stretched), and then when your butt almost reaches the bench, bend your knees and land your feet on the floor. Repeat 5-7 times. When you reach a point where you can no longer bring your legs above your head, do partial reps.

Go up and down with your knees bent. Make sure your butt rises up a couple of inches off the bench on each rep. Do 7-10 reps.

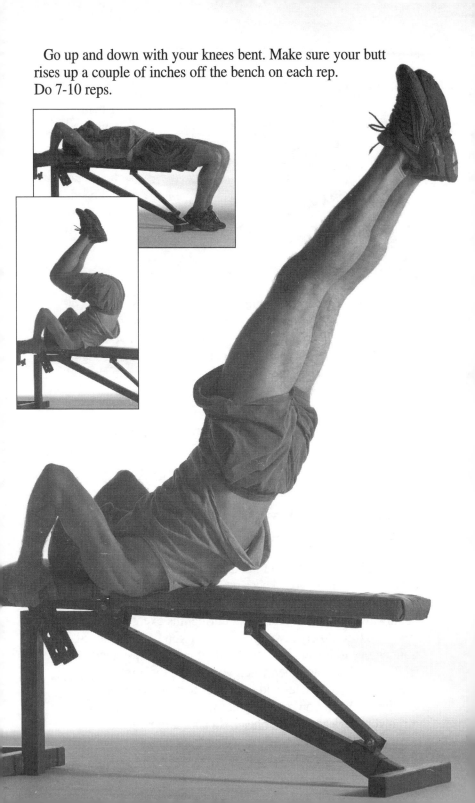

Second Set Crunches: 7-10 reps

When you finish reverse crunches, you'll be in pain.
Nevertheless, you have to go on and do one more set of crunches.

Lie down on the bench and do one
more set of crunches while your legs
are grounded on the floor. Do it the
same way as you did before, for 7-10
reps. By now, you're on fire. All
you'll want is to get out of there. So,
don't wait. Go back to the chin up
bar, grab it, and hang for a couple of
seconds.

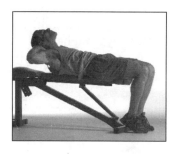

You're almost done with your double cheeseburger. Since we
don't like leftovers, let's finish.

Final Leg Raise

Hang on the chin-up bar with your feet flexed, pointing forward.
With whatever is left within you, bring your feet to eye-level. If
you can't do it with straight legs, do it with your knees bent. Keep
it there for a few seconds, and then slowly bring them down.

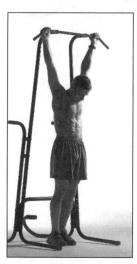

Repeat 5-7 times, or do as many reps as
you can. When you feel the sharp pain on
your rib cage, and on your lower and
upper abs, you can stop pumping. Hang
for a second, stretch your abs, arch your
back ever-so slightly, then stretch your abs
again—and you're all done.

Note: the only way that you can reach
maximum performance with your
midsection is to incorporate lower-back
stretching with ab exercises. The lower
back and abs balance each other. A
weakness in either may create imbalance,
bad posture, injuries, and may compromise
your strength.

Lower-Back Stretch: 1-3 Sets

Lie down flat on your abdominals. Your arms should be straight and at your sides, with your hands palms down to the floor. Your head should be facing forward. With the palms of your hands pushing downward, lift your lower body up. Your legs should be practically straight. Push your lower body up, without jerking, as high as you can. When you reach maximum contraction, hold for 10 full seconds. Relax and repeat again.

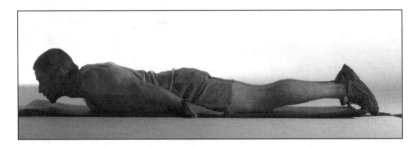

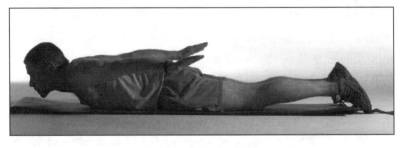

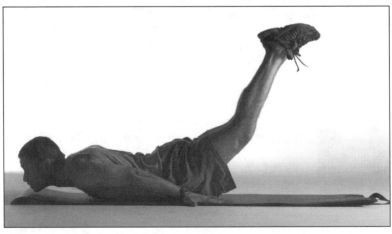

Legs
(Knees, Ankles, Calves, Buttocks, Lower Back)

Leg workouts are based on doing one giant superset, with a few specific pre-exhausting isolation exercises. The goal of these exercises is to activate all the joints involved in leg movements, and to maximize the three factors of strength: intensity, time under pressure, and form. Incorporating pre-exhausting isolation exercises with a giant superset forces your body to train under controlled fatigue. The isolation exercises put maximum pressure on body parts such as calves or hamstrings, which otherwise wouldn't get the maximum intense resistance necessary. Leg workouts are short and intense. They take no more than 15 minutes.

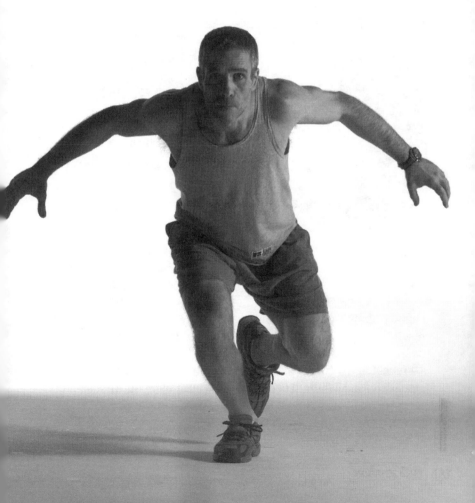

You should train your legs only once a week, to ensure maximum recuperation. If you follow this exercise routine, you'll build strong, lean, functional, very defined legs. You'll also develop your glute muscles and strengthen your lower back.

I generally prefer to use free weights over machines. Free-weight squats, done with the right form, will activate all necessary neuromuscular units and reflexes, which control body balance and movements. Free-weight training activates stabilizing muscles, the small muscles that support the large compound muscle groups. The only way to reach maximum performance is to train all the above muscle groups and take advantage of the synergy between them.

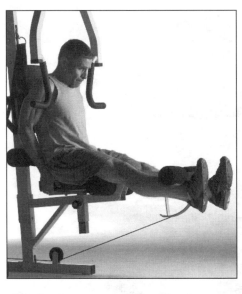

Isolation Exercises

Leg (Knee) Extensions

Declining Set:
1. 8-10 reps, heavy
2. 5-6 reps, medium

Sit on the leg-extension machine. Position your feet under the pad supporting your leg. Adjust the pad to be slightly above your ankle. Slowly extend your legs. When you reach top extension, freeze for a second or two and then slowly bend your knees back to the starting position. Do this again for 8-10 reps. On the fifth rep, try to freeze your leg while fully extended for 5 whole seconds. When you finish your first set, rest for 5 seconds, then, lower the weight, bend your upper body forward and do another set of 5 to 6 reps.

Standing Calf Raises

Declining Set:

1. 10–13 reps, heavy

2. 10 quick reps, medium

You don't need a machine to perform this exercise. However, if you do have access to a machine, it'll enable you to perform more intensely, which will accelerate your strength gain.

Stand with your toes on the attached block on the bottom of the machine. Rest the pads on your shoulders. Lock your knees, keep your legs straight, then move up and down on your toes. When you reach the bottom stretch, stay for one second and then move up to the top flexing position, so your calves are at peak contraction. Then, freeze for one second and go slowly down. Repeat for 10 reps. When you reach the point that you can't go on, do 3–5 half reps. You'll feel the pressure moving from your calves to the stabilizing muscles around and above your ankles. When you finish your first set, rest for 15 seconds. Then, stretch each calf for a few seconds, and then begin your second set. Reduce the weight to the point you'll be able to perform 10 more reps. Do it as quickly as you can—but make sure you keep the right form. The best way to perform quick reps is by counting them (1/2 a second per rep). Your body will follow the rhythm if you count out loud.

Calf Stretching

When you complete this declining set, stretch your calves. While standing in front of the rack, place your toes on the bottom block. The heel of your foot should touch the ground. Bend your knees forward. Make sure that your heels don't leave the ground. The further you bend your knee, the more you stretch your calves.

Standing Calf Raise—
without a machine (One-leg Raise)

Stand on one leg with your toes on a high board or a bench.
Position the bench next to a rack or a door, so that you'll be able
to support yourself with your hand. Go up and down. Stay for one
second on the bottom and for one second on the top. Try to do 15-
20 reps, followed by 3-5 half reps. When you finish one leg set,
change your legs and do the same set with the other leg, only this
time do it facing the opposite direction, so you'll be able to
support your leg with the hand on the same side.

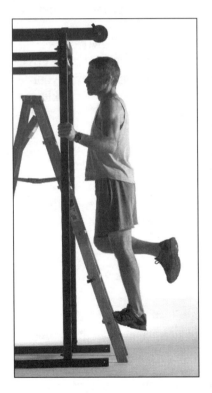
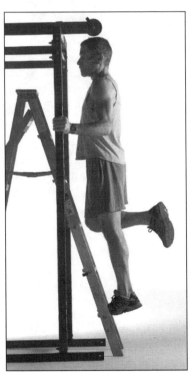

Leg Curls (Hamstrings)

One set for 8–10 reps, heavy

Lie face down on the leg-curl bench. Place your feet under the rollers (the round pad that supports your foot). Curl your legs towards your butt. Make sure that the pad is always touching your butt. When you reach peak contraction, pause at the top and then slowly lower the legs back to the starting position. Repeat again for 8–10 reps. When you do this exercise, make sure that your pelvis doesn't leave the bench. If you have to raise your butt, you're probably using too much weight. Move slowly. To avoid tendon injuries, don't swing or jerk.

Giant Superset

You've just finished some isolation exercises, and have burned your knees, your hamstrings, and your calves. Now it's time to work all leg muscles and joints in one giant superset.

Beginners should choose weights that are light enough to carry all through this superset.

If you're an advanced athlete or bodybuilder, choose a weight that you can squat for 15–20 reps. Don't go too heavy, because you may fail or be forced to compromise on the form. Remember, this is a giant superset. It takes 3-5 minutes, and then you're done. But these few minutes feel like a monstrously long time—so prepare yourself. Within a few weeks, as you become stronger, you can increase the weight or the length of the superset by combining two giant supersets that last about 10 monstrous minutes.

Front Squats

Place the barbell on the squat rack at about shoulder height. Step under the bar and rest it across your front shoulders, just below your chin. Raise your arms straight under the barbell with the palm of your hands pointing up. Cross your forearms and bring them back untilyour hands hold the barbell in an upheld crossed position, your palms above the bar. Slowly pick the barbell up and away from the rack. Step back and place your feet slightly less than shoulder width apart.

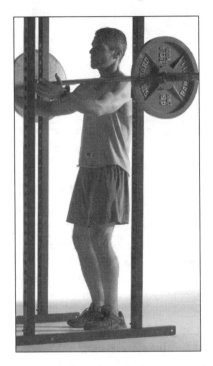 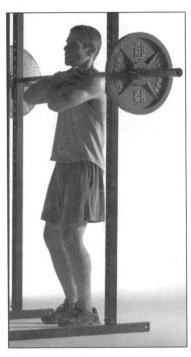

Take a deep breath, keep your back slightly arched, and flex your lower back, which pushes your butt slightly backward. Keep your chin up. Your eyes should stare toward the ceiling. Then, slowly bend your knees and descend toward the floor. Stop when your thighs almost touch your ankles, just below parallel with the floor. Pause for a second, and slowly return to the starting position. Make sure you keep the right form. At all times your back should be arched and your chin should be up. If you feel that the weight pushes you forward and you may lose your balance,

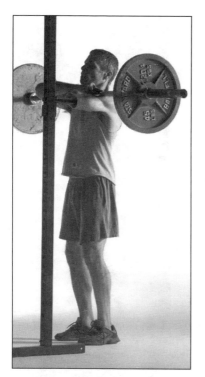
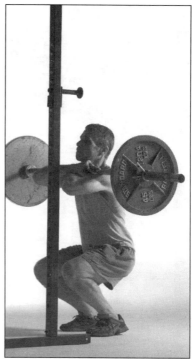

it's a sign that your lower back is weak. Choose a lighter weight so that you'll be able to perform the above routine without compromising the form. Do 8–12 reps.

Back Squats

When you finish, step forward and place the bar back on the rack. Then, take a couple of deep breaths, stay under the bar, and rest it across your trapezius muscles and shoulders. (Your trapezius muscles are located at the top of your middle and upper back. They activate all shoulder shrugs and shoulder blade squeezes.) Step back away from the rack and place your feet about shoulder-width, or slightly more than shoulder-width, apart. Take a deep breath, arch your back, keep your chin up, look upward and slowly decline, bending your knees until your thighs almost touch your ankles. Pause for a second and slowly return to starting position. Repeat again for 8–12 reps.

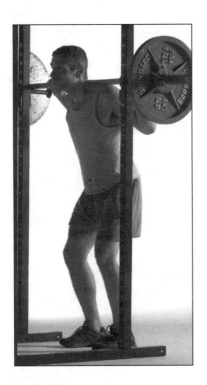

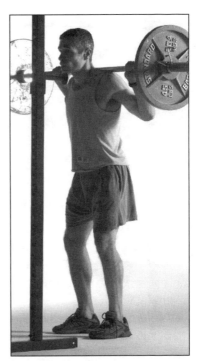

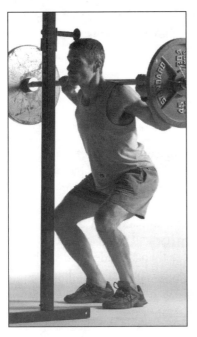

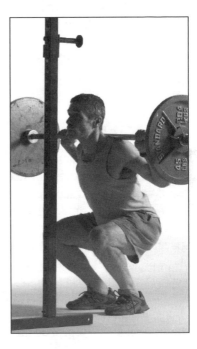

When you've finished, go to the hack squats machine to continue the giant superset. There should be no resting between these sets.

Hack Squats

Place your feet about shoulder-width apart on the machine incline footboard. Your heels should touch the board a few inches ahead of your body. Your toes should point up, not touching the board. Rest the pads on your shoulders. Slowly squat down until your thighs are lower than parallel with the board. Pause for a second, and then return to the starting position. Repeat again. Do 5–6 reps followed by 3–5 half reps from the bottom of the squat position. When you're finished, go back to the squat rack to exercise the last part of the monster superset.

Lunges

Rest the barbell behind your head (the same as for back squats). Lunge one leg in front of the other, about two or so feet apart, keeping the majority of your weight on the front leg. Slowly descend down toward the floor. Pause on the bottom for a second or two, and then slowly rise up. Do 8–10 reps for each leg. When you

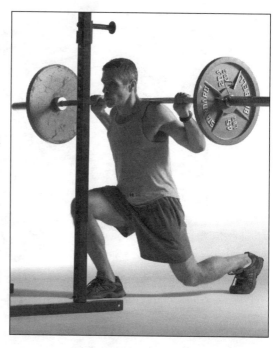

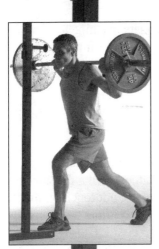

descend toward the floor, make sure that the angle of your front leg is about 90-degrees with the floor.

Congratulations! You've just finished the monster superset.

Now it's time to do some dynamic stretching. The sissy-squats position is a powerful stretch, which will strengthen the muscles and tendons above your knees.

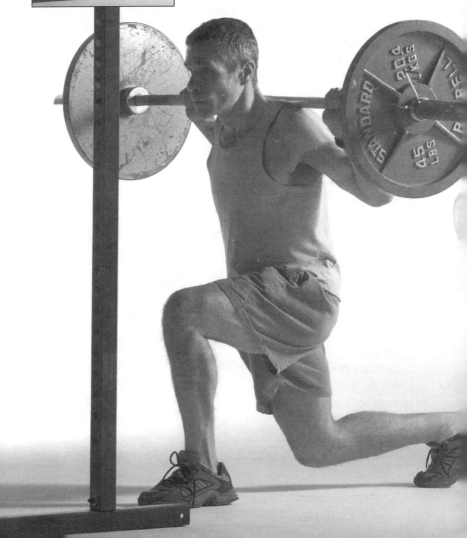

Sissy Squats – Dynamic Stretching

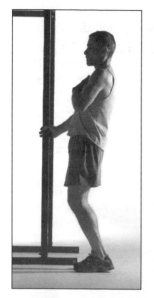
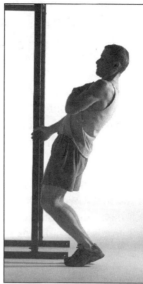

Hold an upright structure for support (wall, rack, or door). Lean your upper body ever so slightly backward, and, with your feet approximately shoulder-width apart, descend to the floor.

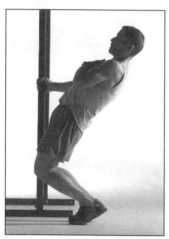
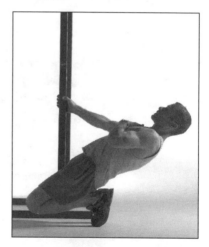

Go down to almost parallel with the floor. Stay for 5 to 15 seconds, and then slowly return to starting position. At all times, keep your back in a straight line with your pelvis—the only thing moving should be your knees. Repeat 3–5 times.

That's all, folks. You can go home now.

Shoulder Exercises

Shoulder exercises are split between two workout days. The reason is that shoulders are relatively small muscles, divided into three groups: front, side, and back. Each muscle group needs maximum attention. By splitting between two days of shoulder workouts, you can concentrate more on each muscle group and be able to apply more intensity to accelerate your strength gain. Conversely, with a one-day shoulder routine, once you exhaust your shoulders with basic press exercises, you may be forced to compromise on the intensity or the form of other exercises, such as laterals or front raises.

Another reason for a two-day-split shoulder workout is the ability to work on the synergy between antagonistic muscles on the second workout day, when you can incorporate raise and pull exercises like side laterals and pull ups.

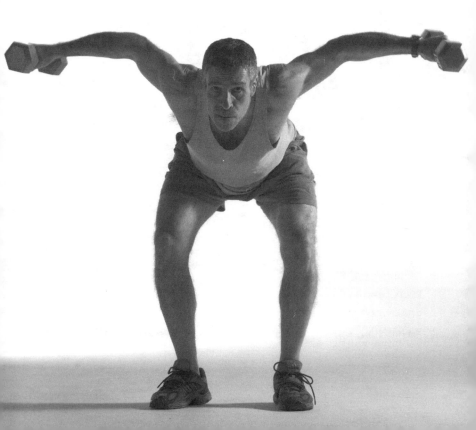

Shoulders—First Day

Shoulder Press/Front Military Press (5 x 5-7)

Sit on the shoulder rack bench. Make sure your mid and lower back are tight. Avoid excess arching. Hold the barbell slightly wider than shoulder width. Pick the barbell off the rack and hold it above your head. Try to feel the weight and say to yourself: "it's a piece of cake." Lower the bar just below your chin, wait for a second, and press it upward to starting position. Repeat this for 5–7 reps. Do 5 sets. You may choose to incorporate two heavy sets of 3 reps (on the second and third set).

Front presses activate all shoulder muscle groups, with an emphasis on front deltoids.

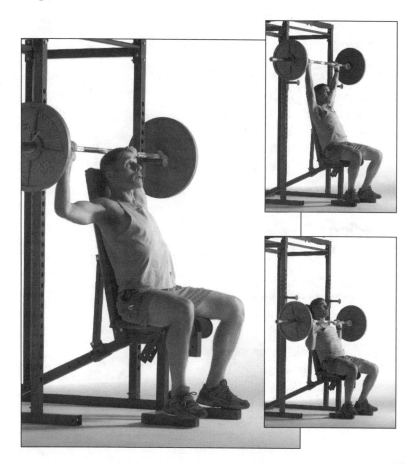

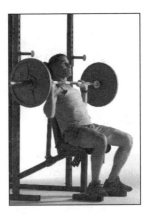

Tendon Stretch

To work on shoulder tendons, finish the above exercise with a special set holding the barbell just above your upper chest for 10 seconds. While you count to 10, push the barbell slightly up on each count. Then, with all your might, press the barbell up above your head and put it back on the rack. For this exercise you might need a spotter to secure the last rep.

Superset:

Standing Barbell Press followed by Front Rows

This superset (1–2 sets) concludes the first day of shoulder exercises. It works all shoulder muscle groups, with an emphasis on shoulder tendons, front and side muscles, and traps.

Standing Barbell Press

Stand above the barbell, with your legs shoulder-width apart. Hold the barbell slightly wider than shoulder width. Bend down, and arch your back. Clean the barbell to shoulder height, just below your chin. Press the barbell above your head, and hold it there

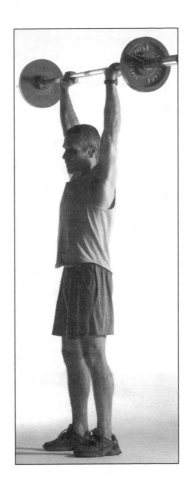

for a second with your arms locked. Keep your abs and lower back tight. Avoid excessive arching. Slowly lower the barbell back to shoulder height. Wait for a second and slowly press the bar again. Repeat for 6–8 reps. When you finish, stand with the barbell resting at shoulder-height, and then slowly lower the bar to arm-length, just below your groin.

Front Row

Start this exercise by narrowing your grip to slightly less than shoulder-width. Lift the barbell up close to the front of your body, until the barbell touches your chin or nose.

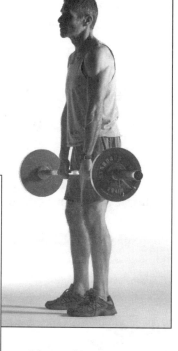

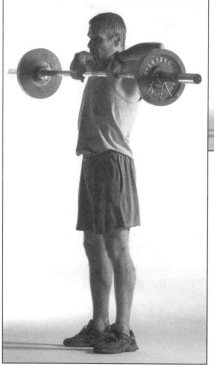

Always keep your elbows pointing to the sides slightly above the barbell. When you reach the top, squeeze. You'll feel the stretch on your sides and the top of your shoulders. The more you squeeze on the top, the more pressure you'll feel on the tendons.

You'll also feel the pressure on your traps. Squeeze for a second or two, and then slowly lower the barbell to starting position. Repeat 5–7 times.

When you reach a point where you can't raise the bar to chin height, use cheat reps. You can lift the bar to chin height by slightly jerking your knees and lower back. Be careful to keep your back arched and your lower back tight. Do not lock your knees. Do 5–7 cheat reps. When you finish, put the barbell on the floor. Do it slowly with arched back (don't jerk), slowly bending your knees until the barbell reaches the floor.

Shoulders—Second Day
Superset: Pull-ups, Shoulder Laterals

The second shoulder-workout day incorporates two giant supersets of shoulder laterals, and front raises with pull-ups. This routine is short and intense. It shouldn't take more than 15 minutes. It works your side and rear delts, your traps, lats, and tendons.

First Superset: Pull-ups, followed by Shoulder Side Laterals and Shoulder Back Laterals

Pull-ups:

Stand under an overhead bar. Most gyms have a special rack for pull-ups, where the overhead bar is marked for wide grip and narrow grip. Grab the bar in a wide grip. Your arms should hang about 45 degrees from your body. Pull yourself up until your upper chest almost touches the bar. Try to keep your back arched all the way up. Stay on the top for a second, and then lower your body back to hanging position. Do as many reps as you can.

When you pull yourself up, keep your chest forward while pushing your body away from the overhead bar. This way you use more of your lats than your biceps.

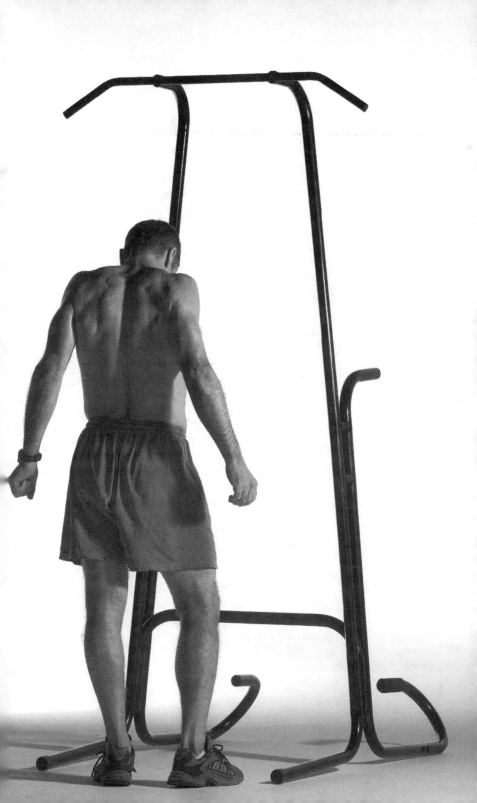

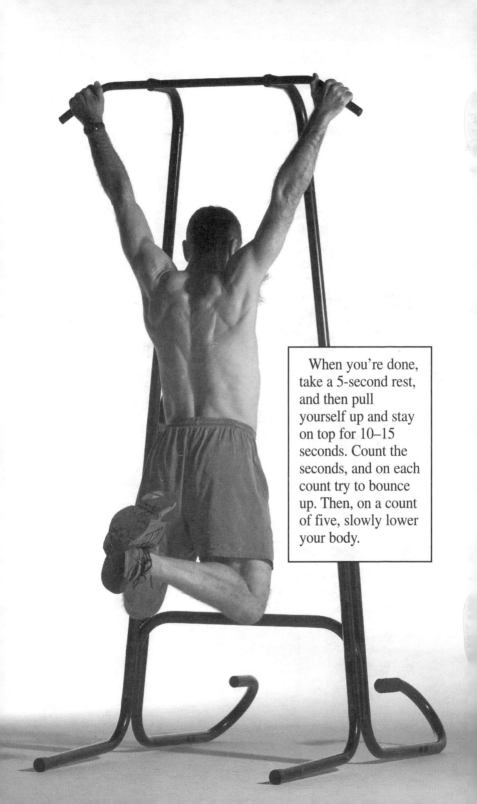

When you're done, take a 5-second rest, and then pull yourself up and stay on top for 10–15 seconds. Count the seconds, and on each count try to bounce up. Then, on a count of five, slowly lower your body.

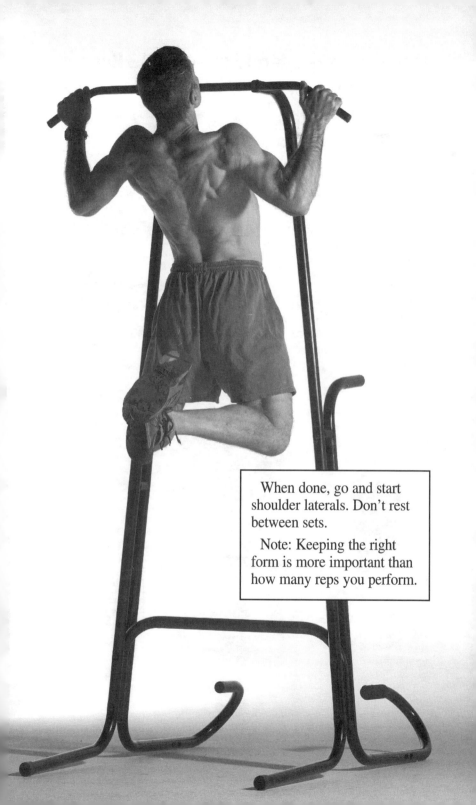

When done, go and start shoulder laterals. Don't rest between sets.

Note: Keeping the right form is more important than how many reps you perform.

Shoulder Side Lateral Raises: 10-13 Reps

Hold the dumbbells by your sides. Bend your elbows slightly. Raise both arms to just a bit higher than shoulder height. While you lift, rotate your hands so that your thumb will be facing downward. When you reach peak contraction, try to hold it for a second. It's going to be hard, but make the attempt nonetheless. Then slowly lower your arms back to starting position. Don't jerk at all. When you're done, start Bent Over Laterals.

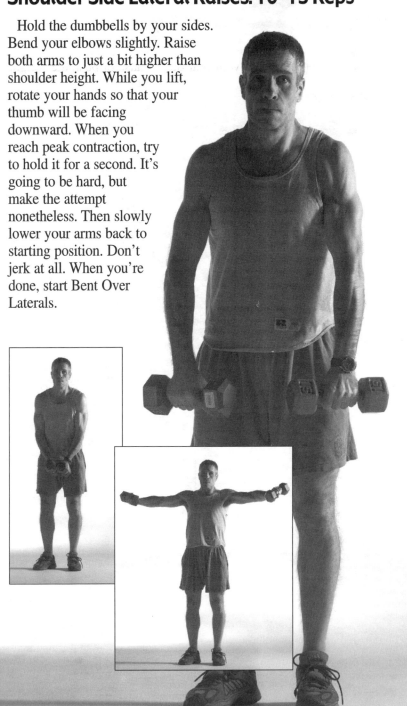

Shoulder Back Laterals—
Bent Over Laterals: 10–15 Reps

This is the same as Side Laterals, only here you bend forward and put more pressure on your rear delts. Raise or push the weight upward. Your hands should be slightly bent. When you feel the burn, you can bend your elbows more and keep pushing the weight up through your rear delts. Do 10–15 reps. When you're done, rest for a couple of minutes, and then start your last exercise for the day.

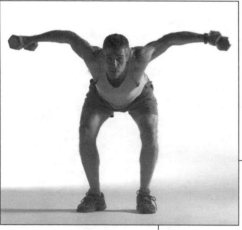

Note: Shoulder back laterals look like a bird taking flight. Think of your arms as wings.

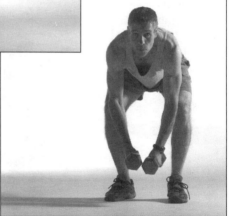

Superset: Pull-ups and Shoulder Barbell Front Raise

This exercise works your lats, biceps, front of the shoulders, and tendons.

Pull-ups: Same as before

Shoulders Barbell Front Raise: 10 Reps

Hold a barbell at shoulder width. Raise the bar slowly above your head. Your arms should be slightly bent at all times. Stay on top for a second, feel the pressure on your tendons, and then slowly lower the weight to starting position. After 5 reps, raise the bar to eye-level, hold it for a second, and then slowly lower the weight. Do 8–10 reps all together. When you're done, grab a lighter barbell. Raise it to eye level. Hold for 5–7 seconds, and then slowly lower the bar.

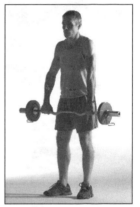

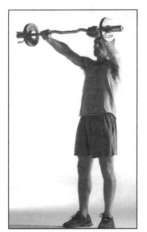

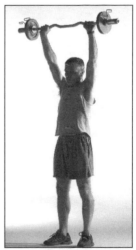

Bow and Arrow—Shoulder Stretch

This stretch routine mimics how ancient warriors used the bow and arrow. It works on the rear delts, back, traps, triceps, elbows, and tendons.

Get yourself a training bungee cord, or, if inaccessible, you can use a towel. Fold the bungee cord. Hold the handles attached to the cord with one hand, and the edge of the folded cord with the other hand. Bring the cord up to shoulder-level. Stretch one hand to the side of your body at shoulder-height, as if you are holding a bow. The stretched hand should be at 90 degrees from your body. The other hand should hold the handles with the elbow bent, as if you are holding an arrow. Slowly pull the string with the bent hand through your shoulder and elbow to the opposite direction of the stretched hand, as if you're about to shoot an arrow. At all times, keep the other hand in a stretched locked position. When you reach peak contraction, stay for 10 seconds. On each second count, slightly pull through your elbow and the shoulder of the pulling hand. Return the pulling hand to starting position. Repeat 5–10 times.

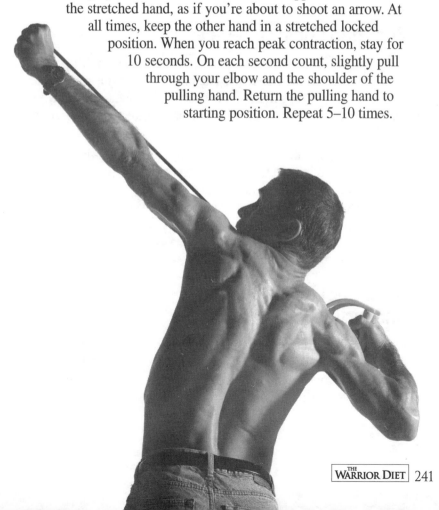

When you're done, change your hand position. The pulling hand should be stretched holding the edge of the folded cord, and the stretched hand holding the handles should be bent. Repeat 5–10 times. At all times, your eyes should stare at the outstretched far hand, as if you're aiming an imaginary arrow at a target.

This completes the shoulder exercises. Take note that you'll work your shoulders somewhat on back and chest days. As mentioned, this is a basic routine that activates all deltoid muscle groups and tendons.

• **Those interested in more information on advanced Warrior Workouts should visit our web site: www.dragondoor.com**

Back and Chest Supersets

Typical bodybuilding exercise routines incorporate pull-ups with back exercises on the same day. The problem with this routine is that by doing pull-ups first, you exhaust yourself and then may be forced to compromise on the intensity of the other back exercises that follow.

The Warrior Workout routine separates between pull-ups and other back exercises. Pull-ups are incorporated, as you know, with shoulder laterals on a separate day, so you can concentrate more on each exercise without compromising your stamina, and the exercise's intensity.

Superset: Lat Pull-downs and Incline Press

This superset incorporates pull and press exercises, taking advantage of the synergy between the antagonistic muscles involved. It works your lats, biceps, triceps, traps, upper back, upper chest, as well as your front delts and tendons.

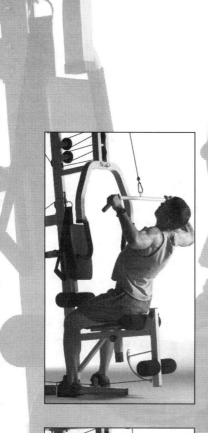

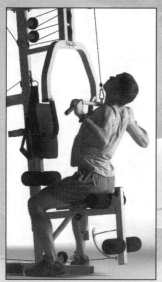

Lat Pull-downs

Sit on the attached pull-down seat.
Hold the bar with a wide grip. Arch
your back. Keep your chin high. Pull
the bar down to the front of your
chest. Pause for a couple of seconds.
Squeeze backward (not downward, as
most people mistakenly do) as hard
as you can. You'll feel your traps and
the lower part of your upper back.
Return slowly to starting position. Do
5–7 heavy reps. Then, lower the
weight. Bend backward until your
back is about 45 degrees to the floor.
Keep your back arched at all times.
Slowly pull the bar to your front
chest. Pause for 5–7 seconds, count
the seconds, and with each count
squeeze the bar toward your chest.
Then, slowly return the bar to starting
position. Do 5 reps. When you're
done, go to the incline chest rack.
Don't rest between sets.

Incline Barbell Press—5 Reps

Sit on the bench attached to the incline rack. If needed, adjust the bench to a 30-degree angle. Pick the barbell up from the rack. Use a grip slightly wider than shoulder width. Most bars are marked for such a grip. Hold the bar, feel the weight. You can say to yourself once again that "this is a piece of cake," even if you don't like cake. Slowly lower the bar to the front of your upper chest. Pause for a second, and press it up above your head. At all times, press your shoulder blades to the bench, slightly arch your lower back, keeping it tight. Do 5 reps. Rest for 10–15 seconds, then grab the bar and slowly lower it to your upper chest. Pause for 5–7 seconds, count the seconds, and with each count bounce the bar away from your body. This will put pressure on your front deltoids and tendons, as well as stretch your upper chest. Then, with all your might, press the bar above your head. You may need a spotter for this last rep.

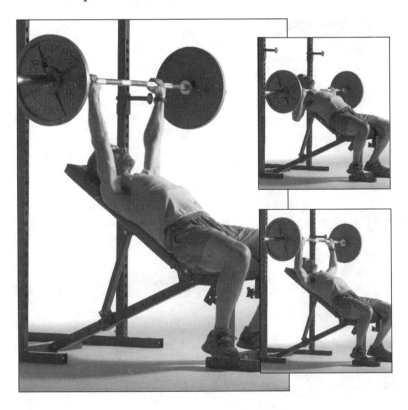

Superset: Seated Pulley Rows and Flat Bench Press

This superset again incorporates push-and-pull exercises by combining antagonistic muscle groups into one set. It works your lower back, middle back, and lats, as well as your biceps, triceps, chest, front deltoids, and tendons.

Seated Pulley Rows— 10 reps, including cheat reps

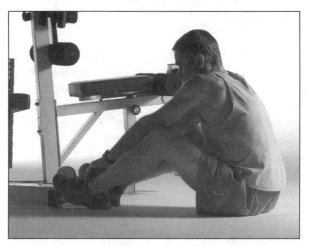

Sit on the pulley rack bench. Bend your knees. Hold the handle or bar attached to the pulley's cable. Arch your back and sit at a 90-degree angle. Pull the bar or handle to your upper abs, just below the chest. Pause for a second. Squeeze and then slowly return to arm stretch (starting position). On the fifth rep, pause at peak contraction for 5–7 seconds. Squeeze the bar to your body on each second count. Then slowly return to arm-stretch position, and bend forward fully stretched.

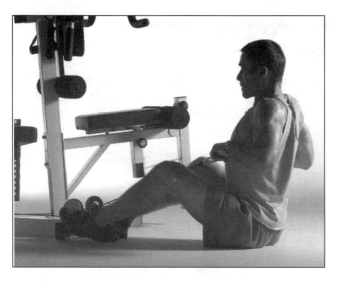

Now you can do a few cheat reps. Pull the bar to your body,
bouncing slightly with your back. Don't bend backward further
than 90 degrees at any time. Bring the bar slowly back to stretch
position. Do 5 cheat reps—for a total of 10 reps. The first 5 slow
reps work your middle and lower back. The last 5 cheat reps
work the lower part of your mid-back, and the sides of your
lower back. When you're done, go to the flat bench rack. Don't
rest between sets.

Flat Bench Barbell Press—5-7 reps

Grab the bar with a wider-than-shoulder-width grip. Most bars
are marked for such a grip. Pick the bar up away from the rack,
and hold it above your chest. Try to feel the weight and say to
yourself, "It's a bitch but I'm gonna do it anyway." Lower the
bar slowly to your mid-chest and then press it back until your
arms are locked out. Do 5–7 reps. When you're done, rest for
10–15 seconds. Then pick the bar up again and slowly lower it to
your chest. Pause for 5–10 seconds. On each second count, push
the bar slightly away from your body. Then, push the bar back to
a locked-arm position. You may need a spotter for this last rep.

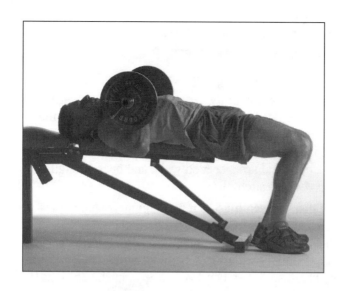

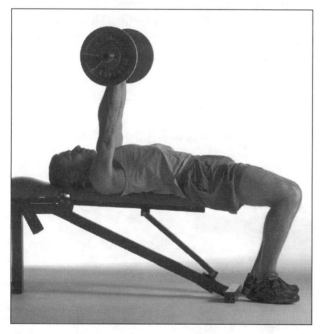

Dead Lifts—1-2 sets, 5-7 reps.
For beginners, 1 set, 10 reps.

This exercise is intense. It works all your body with an emphasis on your lower mid-back, forearms, wrists, knees, calves, waist, and glutes. I consider dead lifts as one exercise that activates the most important compound muscle groups and tendons. It's been written in the Bible that a man's strength is in his waist. Warriors who carried weapons and arms needed waist and back strength. Dead Lifts give you this strength.

Pick a weight that you can lift 5–7 reps. Beginners should pick a light weight to ensure good form. Rest the barbell on the floor. Stand above the bar, your feet positioned just behind the center of the bar, in a stand slightly wider than shoulder-width. Take a couple of deep breaths. Slowly bend your knees, push your butt backward, and at all times keep your back arched while your eyes stare upward. Grab the bar in a slightly wider than shoulder width grip. Hold your breath and slowly pick the bar up from the floor. Your arms should always be locked. Use them as hooks.

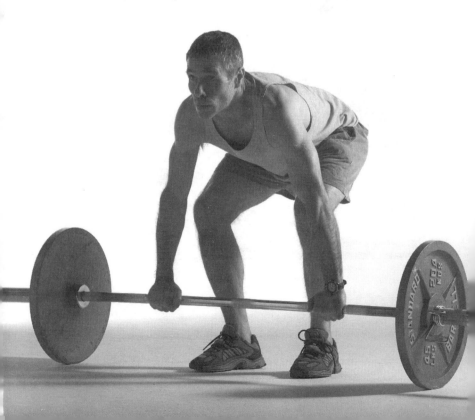

Keep the bar close to the body as you lift and try to maintain a constant arch in your back. Slowly push through your back, butt, knees, and heels, until you are standing straight. When you reach the top, keep your abs and lower back tight. Squeeze your traps, shoulder blades, and buttocks on the top position. Take a deep breath and slowly bend your knees, push your butt backwards, and keep staring upward while your back is arched and tight. Put the bar on the floor. Do 5–7 reps. I like to use a regular grip (hands palm down). This grip will accelerate forearm and wrist strength.

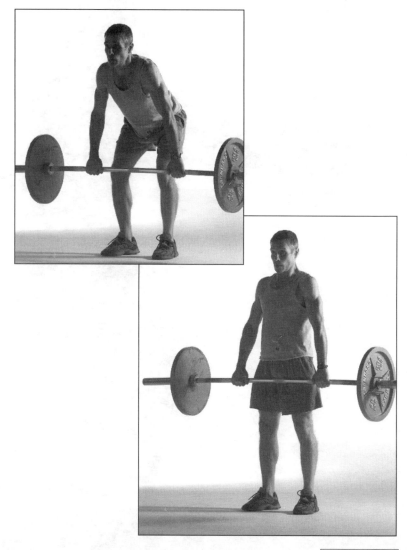

High-Velocity Training: Explosive Exercises

High-velocity exercises can be performed as a one-day-per-week routine. You may choose to incorporate some explosive exercises, such as frog jumps or one-leg jumps, to your daily exercise routine during the week. You can also incorporate high-velocity resistance exercise, such as clean and press, together with intense aerobic exercise, such as sprint intervals to accelerate endurance while training under controlled fatigue.

Clean and Press—3-5 sets, 5 reps

The clean and press is one exercise that works practically all of your body. It's the best exercise for overall muscle synergy, agility, and functional strength. It works your quads, hamstrings, knees, back, traps, shoulders, triceps, biceps, and wrists. If I had to choose only one exercise that would be an effective full-body workout, it would be the clean and press.

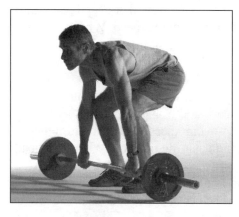

Stand behind the barbell with your feet under the center of the barbell, shoulder-width apart. Bend down and grab the bar with an overhand grip, slightly wider than shoulder width. Keep your back arched and tight, with your eyes staring upward. Take a deep breath. In one explosive motion lift the bar to your shoulders.

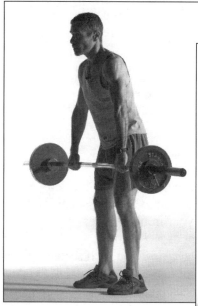

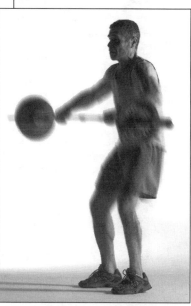

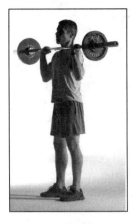

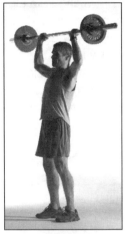

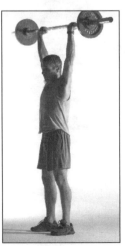

A clean motion in "slow-mo" should look like this: first the bar moves from just above your ankles to knee level. Then, while your butt declines backward, your upper body moves upward, with your arms bending and moving the barbell toward your shoulders. Your knees bounce a little, yet stay slightly bent. At that point, pause for a second, take another deep breath, and press the weight overhead. When you reach the top overhead position, hold for a second. Keep your lower back and abs tight. Stand still. Do not bounce. Then, slowly lower the bar back to your front shoulders, and from here bring it slowly down to your knees, and then return the weight to starting position. When you bend down, always keep your back arched to avoid injury. Repeat 5 times. The weight should be heavy enough, so that you would fail at about 6 or 7 reps. This way you may be able to perform 3–5 repetitive sets of 5 reps with 1 to 2 minutes rest in between.

Those who want to accelerate the intensity of this exercise should consider using the following tips.

Partial-Press Reps

Once you're done with the last rep you can go on and do partial-press reps. Hold the bar on your front shoulders, and then with a count of 5–7 seconds, lift the weight slightly up and down on each second count. Partial reps should be performed on the last two sets.

Clean and Jerk

In the last two sets, once you finish the fifth rep, you can still go on doing two more forced reps of clean and jerk. Once you clean the barbell to your shoulders, slightly jerk through your bent knees and back. The jerk motion will help you to lift the weight overhead. At the top overhead position, hold for a second and then slowly bring the bar back to your shoulders. Bend your knees slightly and then repeat again 2 or 3 times. Clean and press, followed by clean and jerk, will take everything you have. This is one exercise in which you go all out. As noted, it works on strength, endurance, and balance. Incorporating Controlled-fatigue training with clean and press exercises will help you burn fat and accelerate functional strength gain at the same time.

Frog Jumps

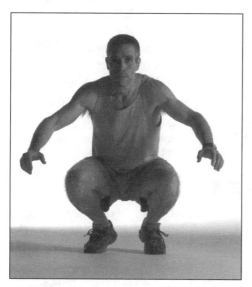

A frog jump is different from a high jump. A frog jump works on the bottom level of a jump-motion range, while a high jump works on the motion's top level. Frog jumps can be performed as a series of jumps forward, sideward, or backward. Ideally, you should combine all these jumps in one set.

This exercise works your knees, calves, ankles, quads, butt, and tendons, with an emphasis on the knees and stabilizing muscles. Frog jumps can be a great warm-up plyometric exercise. It instantly boosts your adrenals, pumping blood all through your body. This exercise will develop your strength, agility, endurance, and balance. However, those who suffer from knee injuries or weak knees should avoid it.

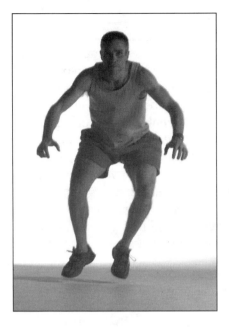

Decline to a squat position, with your back bent forward and your arms slightly bent behind your body. In one explosive motion, lift your body away from the floor while extending your knees. Your arms should move forward and upward while your back extends. Fly as high as you can. It's important to land on the balls of your feet with your knees bent and your back bent and leaning forward. When you reach a squat position, jump again. Repeat 5 times forward, 10 sideward (5 left, 5 right) and 5 times backward. When you finish, rest a minute, and then do another set.

Those people who are in good shape, and want to accelerate the intensity of this exercise, should try to do a few repetitive sets with no rest in between.

Note: Another option for frog jumps is to keep your hands forward or sideward and perform small (low height) but rapid jumps. This means that you jump low and fast in a rhythm of 1-2 seconds per jump. This method will enable you to build volume and endurance.

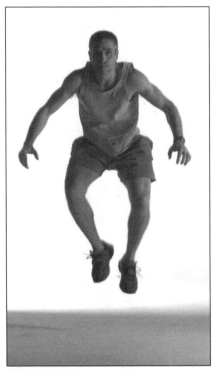

One Leg Jumps: 1-3 sets

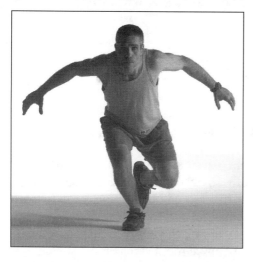

This exercise works on balance, agility, and will develop maximum explosive strength to perform high jumps. It's also a great exercise for building your calves and stabilizing your muscles.

Stand on one leg with the other leg bent slightly, until it feels comfortable. Slowly bend the knee of your standing leg, while

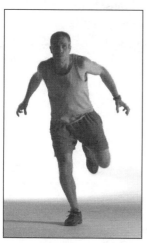

bending your back forward and moving your arms slightly behind you. When your knee reaches an angle of about 45-degrees explode up into the air in one fluid motion while your knee extends, your back bounces up and your arms move forward and upward at the same time. Land on the ball of your foot and explode up again. Repeat 10-20 times for each leg.

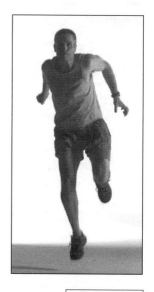

To accelerate the explosive effect of the jump, try to minimize the time your foot touches the ground. It should be like a "touch and go." When you land, it should feel as though you're kicking the floor with the ball of your foot. Do up to 3 sets. You can do one-leg jumps as a warm-up, or else perform jumping sets at the end of your workout.

Those who are interested in more information on advanced high-velocity training should visit our website at **www.dragondoor.com.**

Hamstring Stretches

Standing Hamstring Stretch, 2-3 sets

Stand in front of an upright object, such as a chair, high bench, or a window. Place one leg fully stretched out on the upright object. Your standing leg should be in a locked-out position. Lean forward and try to grab the toes of your elevated foot. Keep both legs fully stretched at all times. If you can't reach your toes, just go as far as you can. When you feel that you've reached maximum stretch, hold the position for 5–10 seconds. To avoid muscle tears, don't press too hard. Relax, go back to starting position, and then do it again. You'll feel the stretch in your hams. Repeat 2–3 times, and then change your legs. Repeat again for 2–3 sets.

Do this stretch after your workout. If you do it before your workout you may hurt yourself and compromise your muscle's ability to contract (by messing up a muscle nerve reflex) since after stretching, the muscle's reflex to contract is compromised.

Biceps and Triceps Superset 1-3 sets

Bicep and tricep exercises are incorporated together in one large superset. They work bi's and tri's, while taking advantage of the synergy between these antagonistic muscles. As you'll soon see, this routine saves time and follows the Warrior Workout principle of keeping the workout short.

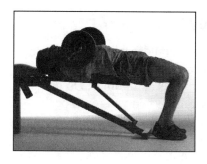

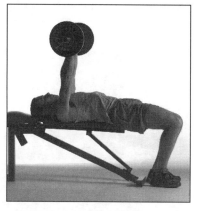

Triceps—Lying Barbell Extensions and Close Grip Presses (tri's and tendons), 5–10 reps

Grab a straight, or an EZ curl bar. Lie down on a flat bench. Position the barbell at arms-locked-out position above your shoulders. Your upper arms should stay still at all times. Bend your elbows, and slowly lower the bar to your forehead. Hold for a second and slowly extend your arms and bring the bar back to a straight-arm position. Repeat 5 times. On the fifth rep, hold the bar above your forehead for 5–7 seconds, and then slowly slide above your face toward your chest. Rest the bar on your chest for a second, and take a deep breath. Press the bar up until you reach the arms-locked-out position. Slowly lower the bar back to your chest. Repeat 5–10 times.

When you're done, grab a barbell heavy enough to do 5–7 reps of bicep standing barbell curls. No resting in between sets.

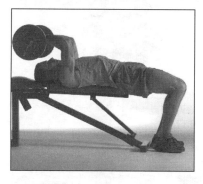

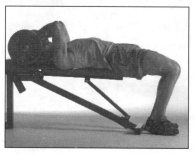

Biceps—Standing Barbell Curls, 5–7 reps

Hold the barbell slightly wider than shoulder-width. With your elbows close to your sides, curl the bar up to about shoulder level. Keep your elbows stationary at your sides at all times. Do not jerk. Keep your back straight. Avoid arching. When you reach peak bicep contraction, slowly lower the bar back to starting position. Repeat 5–7 times. If you're an advanced trainee, you can repeat this superset 1-2 times with no resting in between sets.

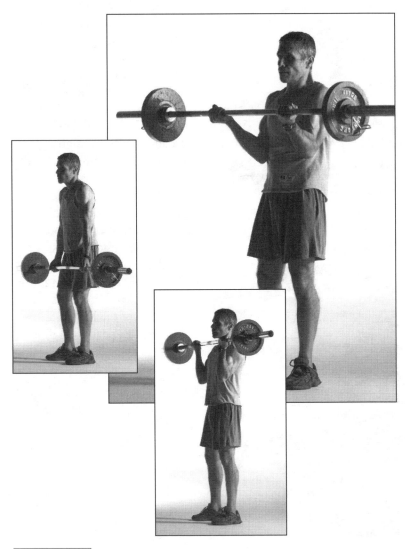

Aerobics

You're probably aware of the benefits of aerobic exercise to your cardiovascular system, mental condition, relaxation, and fat burning. I've found that many people like to separate aerobics from resistance exercises, and I have also observed that even some trainers don't see the synergy between them. Many people who do aerobics for the sole purpose of losing weight skip resistance exercises; conversely, there are those who do resistance exercise only, skipping aerobics.

Warrior Aerobics

Warrior aerobic exercises are specially designed for those who follow the Warrior Workout's controlled-fatigue training routine. I've found that when you incorporate certain aerobic exercises with resistance exercises, it can accelerate functional strength gain and endurance. An added bonus to "mixing things up" is that you should no longer feel stagnated or bored.

Bodybuilders are aware of the fat-burning and toning effects of aerobics, yet many nevertheless look at it suspiciously. Some big guys claim that aerobic exercises like jogging or sprinting places too much pressure on their joints. Others feel that intense aerobics may cannibalize their muscles. Many weekend warriors, who don't have much time to spend in the gym, skip aerobics and do resistance exercises only. People often complain that aerobics are boring, but many continue nevertheless out of guilt due to overindulgence, bad dietary habits, or simply because they've read, or been told by friends or their physician, that twenty minutes of aerobic activity with an elevated heart rate is highly recommended.

Warrior Aerobic Goals

1. Accelerate endurance
2. Improve mental condition
3. Improve speed and agility
4. Burn fat
5. Unleash your instincts

Warrior Aerobic Principles

1. Do aerobics before resistance (as an integral part of controlled-fatigue training)
2. Do it smart. Never get bored.

Warrior Aerobic Exercises

One can do aerobic exercises with different volume, intensity, and form. As noted, those outlined here are the basics.

Aerobics should be done before resistance training. When you do so, your body will begin to adapt and you'll progressively be able to handle prolonged intense pressure more and more easily. Aerobics are an integral part of controlled-fatigue training. As discussed before, your body will instinctively use any resource of energy to generate strength. Granted, this routine isn't easy. However, it pays back generously by making you leaner and tougher.

Let's briefly go over the three factors that affect aerobics: volume, intensity, and form.

Volume: Time under Pressure

The higher the volume, the more calories you'll burn. However, volume alone isn't the only parameter for adapting to prolonged, intense pressure. To illustrate this, there are people who can walk for hours, yet when they try intense exercises such as sprints, they usually collapse after thirty seconds.

Intensity: Amount of Force Generated over Time

Intense aerobics are relatively short in duration. However, short, intense aerobic exercises, such as interval sprints, done progressively, can definitely accelerate endurance and speed, and will enable your body to better handle prolonged intense pressure. An intense aerobic session can be completed in about ten minutes.

Form: Style, Intensity, Speed, Posture, Rhythm, and Balance

Aerobics may be done in different forms, such as walking, jogging, sprinting, swimming, bicycling, jumping, and heavy-bag punching, followed by high-volume resistance training with a short rest in between sets, or a combination of different forms.

Some forms, like heavy-bag punching or sprints, are more intense than, say, slow jogs or walking. As a general rule, the more intense the form, the more your body will be forced to adapt to pressure, and thus, the more strength, speed, and endurance you'll gain.

Intense Aerobics— Sprint Intervals (10–20 minutes)

There are different forms of aerobic intervals. In my opinion, the most practical is sprint intervals since you burn much more energy in a relatively short time than if you had completed a moderate aerobic routine instead. Those who want to accelerate the effect of controlled-fatigue training, without spending much time in the gym, should try sprint intervals. Moreover, it's a progressive method that eventually improves your endurance as well as your strength and speed.

The best way to incorporate sprint intervals in a progressive routine is by gradually increasing their volume and frequency.

Stand on a treadmill. Start on a moderate-tension level. I recommend that you try to run on the balls of your feet. I've found that doing so works like shock absorbers, and lessens the impact on the joints (especially the knees), when compared to the effects I've found running in the traditional heel-to-toe method. Minimize the time that your feet touch the treadmill. Sprint intervals are an explosive form of running, which should eventually improve your speed and strength. In time you'll instinctively improve your style and posture.

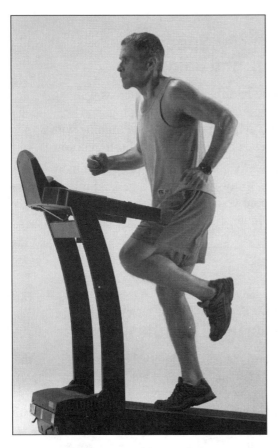

Start running at a comfortable pace. When you've been running for one-and-a-half to two minutes, gradually increase the speed level until you reach the maximum level appropriate for you. Try to sprint for 60 seconds at this level (beginners should start with a 30-second sprint), and then lower it back to where you began, taking 90 seconds to recuperate. Then increase the speed level once again, and do another sprint. Try to incorporate three sprint intervals in a 10-minute run. Advanced trainees should try to increase the last interval to a 90-second sprint.

If there's a mirror in front of the treadmill, look at yourself while you sprint. Always try to improve your posture; make sure that you run forcefully and your feet hit the treadmill in an explosive "touch and go" manner. Your arm movements should dictate the rhythm of your legs and your breathing.

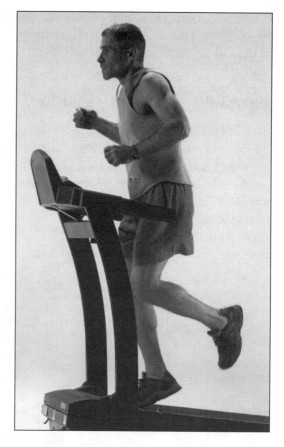

Doing 10-minute sprint intervals is a good way to start. You may feel muscle pain in your calves or sides, and pressure in your joints. Provided you have the right stride and are free of pre-existing conditions (which could hamper your ability to run or appropriateness to do so), you should recuperate and strengthen weak muscles and tendons rather quickly.

From now on everything is open to improvement. You can increase the session to 15 minutes, later to 20 minutes, and can increase the volume of your sprint intervals to 90 or 120 seconds, or increase the frequency of the intervals by shortening the time between sprints.

Don't do this routine every day. You'll need time to recuperate. Start with one session a week, and gradually increase it to two or three times a week. As noted, sprint intervals should be completed before resistance exercises, as part of controlled-fatigue training. It's good to do this routine on leg-workout days, since sprint intervals, combined with leg resistance exercises, are a great way to accelerate muscle development, functional strength, and speed in the most natural and proportional way.

Bicycling/Stationary Biking

• Sprint Intervals

Bicycling places less pressure on your joints than running. Many consider biking a more pleasant and easier way to workout aerobically. In my opinion, whether it's easier or not depends on your level of intensity. You can do sprint intervals when biking in much the same way you do them running.

Start biking on a moderate tension level for four minutes, and then go up to your maximum level, and pump a 60-second sprint. You can also stand on the pedals and push this way until you finish your sprint. Sprint intervals on a bike will improve your strength and endurance. I personally find them less boring than biking on a steady, moderate level.

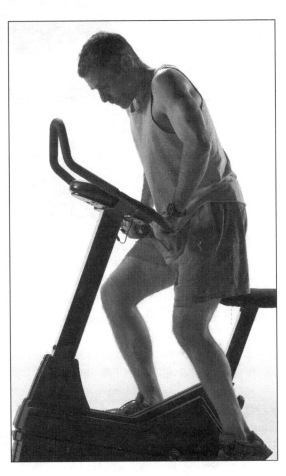

• Reading while Exercising on a Stationary Bike (time well spent)

I find reading while riding is the best way to eliminate boredom. It's also a great way to use your time for studying or learning something. (Well, this depends on what you're reading.) Bring something good to read, and try it if you haven't already. It activates mind and body, which isn't just a slogan. You'll be amazed at how much you can accomplish. I believe that using your brain while you exercise your body improves cognitive functions such as memory and creativity. Don't ask me for research; this is based on my own experience. Reading while riding also makes the time pass much quicker. For those who want to accelerate fat burning through long aerobic sessions, this is a good way to do it.

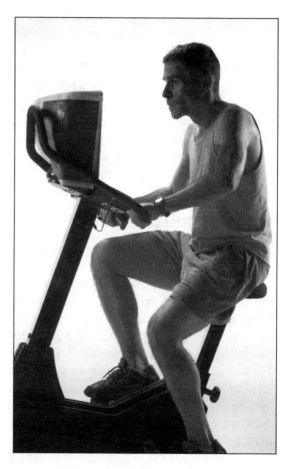

You can choose to alternate between days of biking and days of running, since both methods are good for controlled-fatigue training.

Summary

The Warrior Workout is designed for those who follow the Warrior Diet. The purpose of this workout routine goes beyond losing fat or gaining muscles—it gives you the basis for developing functional strength. Following this exercise routine, you will soon find out that your aesthetic concept of body proportion will compliment your concept of functionality. Most importantly, it helps trigger your Warrior Instinct.

Having a heavy body isn't always a parameter for strength. A human body, first and foremost, is supposed to perform well. From this aspect, being as light and mighty as you can is an advantage. Heavy is okay as long as you're able to effectively run, sprint, and jump. If one of these natural functions is compromised, then something must be wrong. The Warrior Workout trains your body to perform under pressure, while gaining strength, endurance, and agility. It also takes advantage of the synergy between different body movements and muscle groups. Following this routine is a progressive method. You can choose various exercises and combine them according to your personal needs. Follow your instincts. Be creative.

Workout and Diet

It takes some time to adjust to exercising on an empty stomach. I've already discussed the advantages of such a strategy as far as fat-burning efficiency and hormonal manipulation. There is a connection between your last big meal (the night before) and your performance. Those who practice carb depletion (high-protein, low-carbs) may need to reduce the aerobic component of controlled-fatigue training on days following a low-carb diet. Those who practice carb-loading (high-carb meals) will likely find it easier to perform controlled-fatigue training. I recommend cycling between days of low carbs and days of high carbs, and to cycle accordingly short resistance-training days and controlled-fatigue training. I want to mention again how important it is that you use your instincts in planning each workout day. Only you know what's best for you.

Women Who Follow the Warrior Workout

Women are generally smaller than men; they have different needs, and as a result different priorities. Some women may ask themselves, "What do all these workout principles, based on macho-like moves such as slashing, stabbing, swinging, or punching, have to do with me?" The answer to this is that all the exercises outlined in this chapter are essential to create a truly functional body. You may choose to skip these aggressive moves, but why give up the chance to build a truly functional body?

The exercise routine outlined in this chapter mimics the functions of all the above moves without actually doing them. I assume that some women, especially those engaged in martial arts, will have no problem with the Warrior Workout's masculine connotations—or, for that matter, the concept of this book.

My suggestion for women who want to follow the upper-body exercises, such as shoulders, back, chest, and arms, is to make sure to use a weight you can handle all throughout the supersets (which are the core of this routine).

Leg workouts, however, are a different story. Women generally like to work specifically on their legs and buttocks more often than men. I guess this is due to feminine self-awareness, and a desire to keep them in good shape. The Warrior Leg Workout, which is built on a giant superset, places lots of pressure on the lower back and knees. Therefore, I highly suggest women start this routine with no weight.

You can follow all the leg exercises either using nothing at all or by holding a light, wooden stick (like a broomstick). If you use nothing, make sure your hands are positioned as though you're holding an imaginary barbell, and do the repetitions very slowly. When you squat, go down slowly for a count of 5 seconds, then pause for a couple of seconds on the bottom, and then slowly rise up for another count of 5 seconds. You'll be surprised how demanding this is. If you'd like to accelerate the tension on your knees and butt, you can try to freeze, and pause for 10–15 seconds on a slightly higher level than the bottom of your squat.

You can build strong lean and functional legs without using weights. In time, when you feel stronger, you can try to work your legs with light weights.

Regarding all the Warrior Workout exercises listed, my best advice for you is to be creative and use your instincts to design a program that feels right for you.

CHAPTER THIRTEEN
WARRIOR MEALS
AND RECIPES

I'd like to thank Natasha, my wife, for creating some of the Warrior Diet recipes and for improving others. I'm having the fun of my life every night with my family while enjoying these homemade meals.

The Warrior Meals are based on recipes and preparation methods that I use and have continually improved upon since following the Warrior Diet.

For years I've cooked my own meals as part of my daily routine. I've found that when cooking, you treat yourself and those around you with something that satisfies a most basic primal need—nourishment. Cooking is one way of being in control. In my opinion, it's a very human means of showing respect for yourself and your surroundings.

Many of these meals closely mimic old warrior traditions of cooking. The recipes I've included will help you to prepare basic warrior meals. I believe they'll appeal to most people, but since everyone obviously has different tastes, I encourage you to be creative and feel free to tweak them.

I'd like to note up front that you don't have to cook in order to practice the Warrior Diet. Nevertheless, I highly recommend trying it. When you cook your own meals, you become more in tune with yourself and with the food you're eating—and this will enhance your sense of pleasure and satisfaction.

The recipes here are unique to the Warrior Diet. Most aren't available anywhere (that I know of). I haven't explained how to boil eggs, make salads, cook rice, or steam vegetables, since I believe they're common knowledge. Serving sizes and calories per meal are also not included, since they depend on individual needs.

> While reading this chapter, you may realize that some traditional ethnic dishes, such as bouillabaisse, paella, gumbo, and stews closely resemble traditional warrior meals.

Meats

I often cook meat, such as chicken breast, veal, and fish, in a way that mimics the ancient warrior tradition of cooking—in broth—with different herbs and spices to enhance flavor and aroma. Those listed here are my personal favorites. I eat them almost every day, rotating between chicken, veal, and fish.

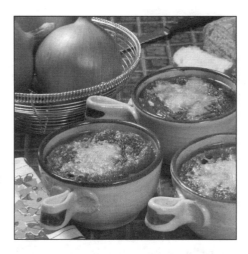

As noted in the "Overeating Phase" and "Lessons from History" chapters, cooking meats in liquids is healthier than frying, grilling, or even baking. Moreover, when cooking in liquids, the meat becomes soft and tender, while absorbing all the flavors of the herbs, spices, and veggies in the broth.

When these meals are fully cooked, I like to shred the meat with a fork and then add some essential oil and lecithin on top. You then get a soft, mushy, delicious protein meal, which hopefully will provide much pleasure as well as health—the old-fashioned way.

> I like to add essential oils and lecithin on top of my meals just before eating. It enriches the nutritional composition of the food and, in my opinion, enhances flavor. Some people, however, may find their taste too strong. Although adding essential fatty acids (EFA) and lecithin are optional, they are nonetheless essential to have in your diet, especially the EFA.

Curry Chicken in Spicy Tomato Broth

Ingredients:

1 ¹/₂ lb. of boneless, skinless chicken breast, cut into medium sized chunks

1 can of stewed tomatoes, chopped (or crushed tomatoes)

1 can of fat-free chicken broth

3 cloves of garlic

¹/₂ small onion

1 bay leaf

1 tablespoon of curry powder

1 tablespoon of turmeric powder

1 tablespoon of dried parsley

³/₄ teaspoon of dried basil

³/₄ teaspoon of dried oregano

³/₄ teaspoon of dried cumin

¹/₄ teaspoon of ground coriander

Salt and pepper to taste

Garnish with ¹/₂ cup of coarsely chopped cilantro

Preparation:

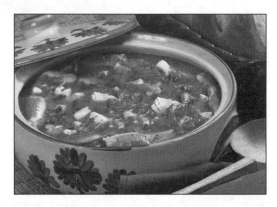

Clean and wash chicken with filtered water. In a large Pyrex bowl (with oven-safe cover) mix all ingredients, excluding the cilantro. Marinate chicken in the bowl (with cover on) overnight in the refrigerator. Marinating overnight is optional.

Preheat oven to 375° F. Cook for one hour in a Pyrex bowl with an oven-safe cover. Serve garnished with chopped cilantro.

This meal goes very well with steamed carrots, zucchini, and broccoli. Starches that most complement this meal are mashed butternut squash, pumpkin, sweet potatoes, mashed potatoes, sweet yellow corn, and rice.

Fish and Eggplant in Curry Tomato Sauce

The Warrior Fish and Eggplant Meal may greatly benefit those people interested in rapid weight loss.

Ingredients:

1 1/2 lb. of white fish fillet (sole, flounder, turbot)
1 can diced or crushed tomatoes (14.5 oz.)
2 medium or large eggplants, peeled and cut into medium size chunks
1 tablespoon olive oil
3 cloves of garlic
1/2 small onion (optional)
1 tablespoon curry powder
1 tablespoon caraway seeds (optional)
3/4 teaspoon oregano
3/4 teaspoon thyme
Salt and cayenne pepper to taste (optional)
1/2 cup chopped fresh cilantro or parsley for garnish

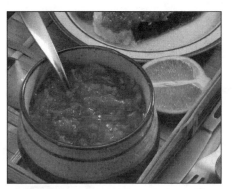

Prepare the sauce in a large Pyrex bowl (with cover) mix all ingredients excluding the cilantro, parsley, and eggplant.

Preparation:

Clean and wash the fish fillet with filtered or spring water.

Place the eggplant chunks in a steamer and cook until they are soft (about 15 minutes).

Marinate the fish in the Pyrex bowl with the sauce.

Preheat oven to 375° F. and cook the fish in the sauce for one hour. When done, remove from oven, add the steamed eggplant, and mash it all together with a fork.
Garnish with chopped, fresh cilantro or parsley.

This meal also mimics an old tradition of warrior cooking. You'll be surprised how big this dish looks; however, it's very light and delicious. Fish meals go very well with steamed carrots, broccoli, cauliflower, rice, millet, and corn.

Veal and Carrots in Chicken-Tomato Broth

Ingredients:

1 ¹/₂ lb. of trimmed veal scallopini, cut into medium chunks
1 large peeled carrots, cut into small medallions
1 can of crushed tomatoes or tomato sauce
1 can of fat-free chicken broth
3 cloves of garlic
¹/₂ onion
1 teaspoon dried basil
³/₄ teaspoon dried oregano
1 tablespoon caraway seeds (optional)
Coarsely chopped parsley or cilantro as garnish

Preparation:

Clean and wash veal with filtered or spring water. If you want the veal to be more tender, beat it with the bottom of one of your cooking pans. No joke! It'll make it softer and absorb more flavor from the broth.

In a large Pyrex bowl, mix all ingredients, excluding the parsley (or cilantro)

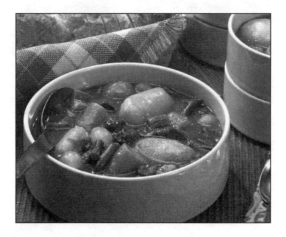

Marinate the veal overnight in the refrigerator (optional)

Preheat oven to 375° F. and cook for 1¹/₂ hours

Garnish with chopped parsley or cilantro

This meal goes very well with steamed broccoli, cauliflower, and zucchini, and for starches, mashed potatoes, mashed butternut squash, and sweet potatoes.

Eggs

Most egg meals take almost no time to prepare and cook, yet they're delicious and very nourishing. On days that I'm too busy, or just in the mood for a light protein meal, eggs are the perfect alternative to meat or fish. Moreover, on egg days I like to indulge every once in a while with dairy foods as well. I think eggs and cheese complement each other nicely.

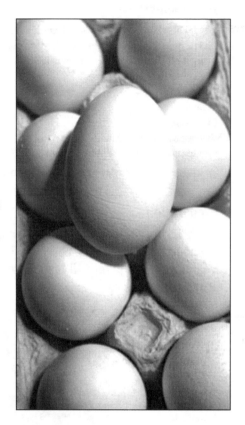

Egg meals can be designed as high-protein meals or as high-carbohydrate meals.

Egg-White Omelet with Tomato Sauce (high protein meal)

Ingredients:

16 egg whites with 3–4 yolks

1/4 cup of tomato sauce or crushed tomatoes

1/4 small onion, diced (optional)

1 tablespoon olive oil

Salt and cayenne pepper to taste

Garnish with chopped parsley or cilantro

Preparation:

Preheat olive oil in a large, deep skillet.

Add diced onions and sear until browned.

Slowly add tomato sauce, mix with onions.

When sauce is boiling, add the eggs.

Scramble and mix the eggs while cooking.

When mixture thickens, remove from the stove, put in a large bowl and cover.

Garnish with the chopped parsley or cilantro.

Those people who like mushrooms can steam shiitake or Portabella mushrooms, or sauté them in olive oil, and put them on top of the omelet. Or you can cook them with the omelet.

Egg omelets go very well with steamed zucchini, butternut squash, steamed pumpkin, sweet peas, and black bean soup, which you can also put on top of the omelet.

Egg-White Omelet with Black Beans (high protein meal)

This is the same preparation as the egg-white omelet with tomato sauce, only here you use black bean soup instead of tomato sauce. You can use a 1/2 can of organic black bean soup, which is available in most health-food stores and supermarkets.

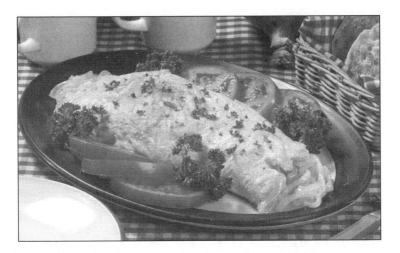

Egg White Omelet with Lentil and Bean Chili (high protein meal)

This is the same preparation as the other omelets, only here you use a 1/2 can of organic chili, which is available in most health-food stores and supermarkets.

Oatmeal and Eggs (high carbohydrate meal)

I used to eat this meal years ago, when I was a student. This was one of my so-called "poor man" meals, since my budget at that time was very limited. Regardless, I always enjoyed it, and still do.

Ingredients:

2-3 cups oatmeal (rolled oats or steel-cut oats)

6-12 egg whites with 2-4 yolks

1/4 teaspoon turmeric (optional)

1/4 teaspoon cumin (optional)

Salt and pepper to taste

1/2 cup coarsely chopped cilantro for garnish

Preparation:

If you choose steel-cut oats, soak them overnight in purified, steam-distilled or spring water (to cut down on cooking time).

In a large pot, fill 4–5 cups water and bring to a boil.

Add oatmeal and spices. Rolled oats need half the time that steel-cut oats need. Check the preparation instructions on the box.

Reduce heat and let it cook until almost done. Make sure you mix it, to avoid clumping. When you notice that very little water is left, add the eggs and slowly mix it all together while still cooking. Once the eggs are thickening, turn the stove off, cover, and let it simmer for a couple of minutes.

Garnish with cilantro and serve.

This meal goes very well with buttermilk or kefir, which will supply additional protein to this high-carbohydrate meal, as well as beneficial bacteria. They can be used as a cool sauce you put on top. Oatmeal and eggs also go well with steamed broccoli and cauliflower.

If you'd like to make this dish spicy you can add curry or cumin. It can also be garnished with scallions or chopped onions. Use your imagination. With trial and error, you'll find what's best for you.

Rice 'n' Eggs
(high carbohydrate meal)

This was my second favorite meal during my student days. Once you taste it, you'll realize that a poor man's meal isn't necessarily poor. It is, in fact, rich in flavor, delicious, and very nourishing.

Ingredients:

2 cups uncooked brown rice, or, if accessible, sweet brown rice. If you prefer, use white rice instead (sushi rice is best).

1 clove chopped garlic

$1/2$ teaspoon curry

$1/2$ teaspoon cumin

$1/2$ teaspoon basil

6-12 egg whites and 2-4 yolks

Chopped cilantro, onions or scallions as garnish

Preparation:

Rinse the rice with purified water. In a large pot, add 4 cups of water with the garlic and spices. Bring to a boil. Stir in the rice, reduce heat, cover and simmer until water is almost absorbed. Add the eggs and mix it with the rice while it's still cooking. When the eggs start to thicken with the mixture, remove from the stove, cover, and let sit for a few minutes. Garnish with cilantro, onions, or scallions and serve.

This meal goes very well with cucumber and dill salad. It also goes well with black bean soup that can be used as a sauce on top of the meal. Those who like to experiment can try grated Parmesan cheese on top, or goat cheese as a side dish.

Angel Hair Rice Pasta with Eggs (high carbohydrate meal)

Ingredients:

1 package of angel hair rice pasta

$1/2$ to 1 can of tomato sauce

2 cloves crushed garlic

$3/4$ teaspoon dried basil

$3/4$ teaspoon dried oregano

6-12 egg whites and 2-4 yolks

Salt and pepper to taste

Parsley or cilantro as garnish

Preparation:

Cook pasta until done. Drain and place the pasta in a large bowl. Mix tomato sauce, garlic, and spices in a large pot and cook on medium-high heat. Add pasta. When hot, add the eggs and mix it all together. When eggs start to thicken, remove from the stove and serve, garnished with cilantro.

You can opt to prepare pasta and eggs without the tomato. In this case, use olive oil as a base to simmer the pasta and eggs in a large, deep pan or pot. Pasta and eggs, done without tomatoes, can be served with buttermilk or kefir as a cool sauce on top of this hot meal. It also goes very well with steamed carrots, zucchini, or broccoli.

If you'd like to increase the amount of protein in this meal, you can add low-fat, organic cottage cheese on the side, or goat cheese on top.

Baked and Grilled Meals

Once in a while, especially when friends are coming over, my wife prepares grilled meats or fish. These meals are more than delicious. They're awesome. Grilling isn't the preferred way to cook on a daily basis. However, when you marinate meats before grilling you reduce the risk of burning or caramelizing the protein. Further, adding herbs like basil, oregano, and thyme, in addition to improving taste, mimics an old tradition of curing meats while enhancing flavors.

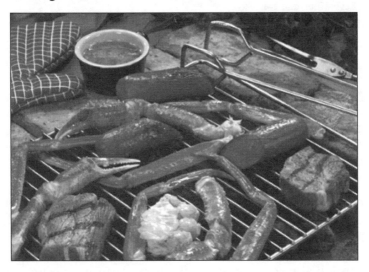

Most herbs contain healing properties. For instance, thyme and oregano are believed to have antibacterial and antiviral properties, turmeric is a powerful antioxidant, and as discussed earlier, parsley is a powerful detoxifier.

Grilled Chicken

Ingredients:

2 packages of boneless skinless chicken thighs
Juice of two lemons
3 large cloves of garlic
1 small onion
1 tablespoon Dijon mustard
1 tablespoon fresh thyme (leaves only, not the stem)
1 tablespoon fresh oregano
1 tablespoon fresh parsley
2 tablespoons fresh basil
3 tablespoons olive oil
Salt and pepper to taste

Preparation:

Combine garlic, onion, mustard, thyme, oregano, parsley, basil, and olive oil in a food processor. Pulse until all ingredients are finely chopped. Season with salt and pepper to taste. Set aside in the fridge for approximately 45 minutes to an hour.

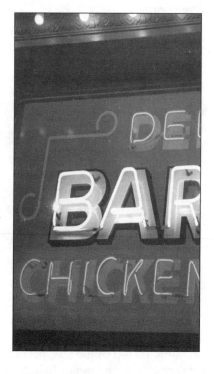

To prepare the chicken for outdoor grilling:

Wash and clean chicken thoroughly. In a bowl combine lemon juice and the mustard mixture with the chicken. Mix well. Let it sit in the fridge for 30 minutes, or until ready to grill. If you don't want to grill, the broiler works fine, too. Grill for approximately 15 minutes on each side on a low to medium flame (check sooner if you're broiling). Just make sure the chicken juices run clear.

Baked Red Snapper

Ingredients:

1 medium whole red snapper
2 large onions, sliced
3 ripe tomatoes sliced
5 lemons
4 cloves of garlic, finely chopped
3 tablespoons olive oil
Salt and pepper to taste

Preparation:

Make sure the fish is properly cleaned of all scales.
Preheat oven to 375° F.

Place ⅓ of the onion and tomato slices on the bottom of a baking pan. Sprinkle a portion of the garlic on the onion and tomatoes. Squeeze the juice of one 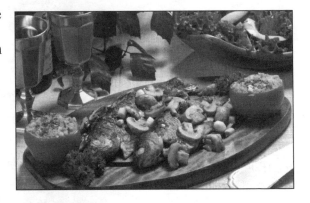 lemon. Before placing fish on the onion and tomatoes, rub fish with salt and pepper. Stuff ⅓ of the onion, tomato, and garlic inside the belly of the snapper. Place the remaining onion, tomato, and garlic on top of the snapper. Take one lemon; cut into slices and spread over the top of fish. Squeeze the remaining lemon on top of the fish. Drizzle olive oil over the fish. Cover with aluminum foil. Cook for 40--50 minutes (depending on the size of the fish).

To test for doneness:

Poke fish with a fork—the meat should be flaky.

Soups

Soups are wonderful appetizers. In addition to introducing different tastes, smells, textures, and aromas, they can be very nutritious and nourishing. Having a soup at the beginning of a meal will enhance your feeling of satisfaction. Soups can also be the basis for a whole meal. As noted, by adding meat, fish, or eggs with beans, and occasionally with carbs such as potatoes, rice, or barley into the broth, you can create a whole, delicious, nutritious meal in the old, traditional way.

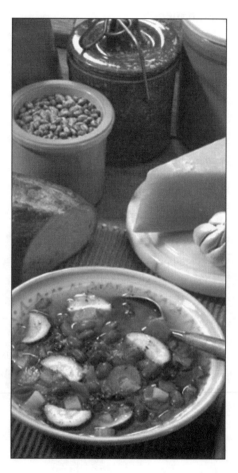

Potato-Onion Tomato Soup

Ingredients:

2 lbs. potatoes, peeled and cut into chunks
1 35-oz. can plum tomatoes with juice, coarsely chopped (total of 4 cups)
1 qt. chicken stock
1/2 teaspoon coarse sea salt
1/4 teaspoon freshly ground black pepper
3 tablespoons extra virgin olive oil
4 medium onions, thinly sliced

Preparation:

In a four-to six-quart non-aluminum saucepan, combine the potatoes, tomatoes, and chicken stock. Season with salt and pepper. Bring to a boil, then reduce heat and simmer gently, partly covered. Stir occasionally, for one-and-a-half hours, or until tender.

Meanwhile, in a skillet, warm olive oil over medium heat and sauté the onions until translucent.

To finish soup, break up potatoes, mashing slightly with a wooden spoon. Add onions to tomato/potato mixture, and simmer together for five minutes, stirring occasionally. Add chicken stock as necessary to slightly thin out the soup. Garnish and serve with fresh basil.

Miso Soup

Miso is made from unpasteurized fermented soybeans. Miso soup is high in minerals and is a wonderful alkalizer. Miso, unlike processed soy foods, is also believed to be a very nutritious food, which can protect against radioactive pollution. It's rich in enzymes and lactic-acid producing bacteria—which is highly beneficial for digestion and elimination.

Ingredients:

1 tablespoon of miso paste (from organic unpasteurized fermented soy)
1/2 small onion
1/2 oz. dried wakame or nori seaweed (optional)
2 cups purified or spring water

Preparation:

In a medium pot, combine all ingredients.

Bring to a boil for 5 minutes.

Serve warm.

Miso Meals (shellfish, fish, or meats):

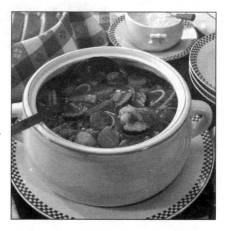

You can opt to add seafood or chunks of fish to the soup, but then you've got to let it cook for 30–45 minutes. If you use miso as a base for a whole meal, taste it to determine whether it's too salty. If so, add more water. Miso is high in enzymes, so when marinating fish or seafood with miso, it'll make the meat more tender.

Desserts

The Warrior Desserts can be great alternatives to sugar-loaded, high in saturated fat, commercial or homemade treats.

There aren't many desserts listed here. However, in my opinion, you'll be better off enjoying the taste of a few healthy delicious desserts that will nourish and give you a great sense of pleasure and satisfaction, than trying a variety of popular desserts and sweets which usually leave you sluggish, bloated, and heavier, not to mention the obvious guilt.

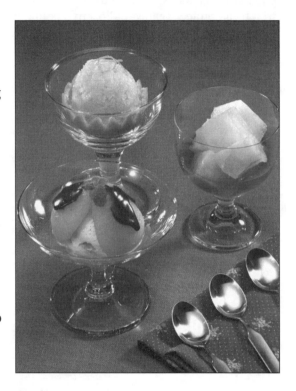

Pumpkin Cheesecake

Ingredients:

1 teaspoon ground cinnamon
1/2 teaspoon ground ginger
1/4 teaspoon ground cloves
Pinch of salt (optional)
1/2 teaspoon vanilla extract
2 whole eggs
4 egg whites
1/4 to 1/2 cup of maple syrup (adjust sweetness according to taste)
1 15-oz. can of organic pumpkin
15 oz. nonfat ricotta cheese (or farmer cheese)
4 oz. fat-free cream cheese

You can substitute these cheeses with organic, low-fat cottage cheese. However, this will change the texture of the cake slightly.

Preparation:

Combine cinnamon, ginger, cloves, and salt (optional) in a small bowl. Set aside. Lightly beat vanilla, eggs, and maple syrup in a small bowl. Set aside. In a food processor, combine pumpkin and cheese until smooth. Add, alternating egg mixture and spice mixture, to the pumpkin and cheese mixture. (If you don't have a food processor, a blender will work, but mix eggs first, then gradually add pumpkin mixture.)

Mix well, approximately three minutes. Bake in a preheated 425 o F. oven for 15 minutes. Reduce temperature to 350 o F. Bake for 40--50 minutes or until a knife inserted near the center comes out clean. Cool and rack for about two hours. Serve room temperature or chilled. Do not freeze; freezing causes the filling to separate.

Pumpkin cheesecake tastes so good that, unfortunately, it disappears too quickly. It's like an open invitation for a binge.

The sweetness can be adjusted according to your taste. It goes very well with organic yogurt or low-fat sour cream. As you can see, this dessert is high in protein, low in fat, and relatively low in carbs. It's also highly nutritious, supplying you with abundant

Crepe Blintzes

Ingredients:

1 egg
8 oz. low-fat cottage cheese (small curds)
1 teaspoon vanilla extract
Pure maple syrup to taste
1 package prepared crepes
Cooking spray (butter-flavored)

Preparation:

Preheat oven to 350° F.

Combine cottage cheese, egg, vanilla, and maple syrup in a small bowl. Take individual crepe, place on a flat surface, spoon one-and-a-half tablespoons of cottage cheese onto center. Fold all four sides together to secure cottage cheese mixture.

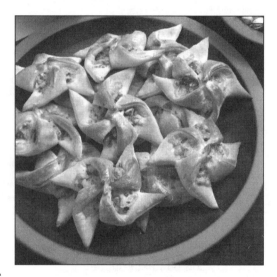

Place each crepe on a nonstick cookie sheet, folded side down. Repeat until cottage cheese mixture is finished. Spray each crepe with butter-flavored spray. Bake in oven for five to eight minutes, until slightly brown. Serve warm with Live Berries.

Live Berries Dessert

Ingredients:

1 cup blackberries
1 cup sliced strawberries
1 cup raspberries
1 cinnamon stick
Pure maple syrup to taste
Sweet red wine
(enough to cover berries)

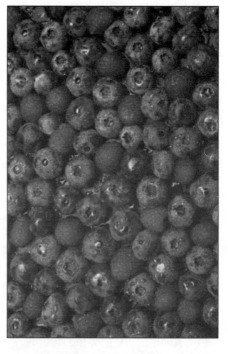

Preparation:

Combine all ingredients in a small bowl and place in fridge for three to four hours to chill (may remain in fridge overnight).

Serve over warm, crepe blintzes.

Suggestion: Live Berries can also be served over yogurt.

This is a meal with total appeal: a feast that screams calories but really is a bounty of low fat, low-cal goodness.
Enjoy!

Milk Gelatin Dessert

I began making this treat years ago. Surprisingly it's turned out to be one of my favorites. Milk Gelatin is a good complement to the fruits and veggies you consume during the day while you go through the Undereating Phase. It's most useful to eat this on an empty stomach.

Ingredients:

1-2 tablespoons of organic nonfat milk powder

1-2 teaspoon of brown rice syrup (adjust sweetness according to taste)

1 packet of unflavored (if available, kosher vegetarian) gelatin

1-2 cups filtered or spring water. Check instructions on the box, but feel free to alter depending on level of intensity desired.

3 tablespoons cool or cold water

2 tablespoons hot water

Vanilla extract to taste (approx. 1/8 teaspoon)

Approximately 3–10 crushed organic almonds (optional)

1–2 tablespoons minced, organic, unsulfured unsweetened coconut (optional)

Preparation:

In a small bowl, mix the milk powder, brown rice syrup, and 1 tablespoon of cool water until it turns into a thick paste. Set aside.

To prepare gelatin:

Mix gelatin in another small bowl with 2 tablespoons of cool or cold water. When it turns into a gummy paste, add 2 more tablespoons of hot water and mix. Combine gelatin mixture with milk paste and then place it in a blender with 2 cups of water. Blend for one minute. Pour mixture into several cups or one large bowl. Refrigerate for a couple of hours until it turns into gelatin form.

You can opt to add more milk powder to make it thicker or more intense. You can also blend a few crushed almonds with the mixture if you want to add texture. And, you can do the same with minced coconut, or else sprinkle it on top once you've poured the completed mixture into a bowl or cups. When it's ready, Milk Gelatin becomes a three-layered treat with a light, white foam on top. It's quite unique. I hope you'll like it.

Papaya Gelatin Dessert

This dessert is good for digestion and detoxification. It can also be consumed as a delicious light treat during the Undereating Phase. Gelatin is a natural source of silicon and glycans, which support your skin, hair, nails, and connective tissues. It's also a great detoxifying agent. Papaya contains digestive enzymes. When eaten on an empty stomach, Papaya Gelatin Dessert soothes your hunger while helping to eliminate toxins, fat, and cholesterol from your intestines.

Ingredients:

1 packet of unflavored (if available, kosher vegetarian) gelatin, which is equivalent to 1 level tablespoon

1 cup of papaya puree (no sugar added). This is sold in glass juice bottles in some health food stores and supermarkets. Or you can puree a fresh papaya yourself. Peel, remove seeds, and cut papaya. Place papaya slices in a blender with a little water and blend until pureed.

1/2 cup hot water (filtered or spring water)

3 tablespoons cool or cold water

2 tablespoons hot water

1 teaspoon of maple syrup (optional)

1 tablespoon minced organic unsulfured, unsweetened coconut (optional)

Preparation:

Heat water on stove. Meanwhile, mix gelatin with 2 tablespoons of cool or cold water in a small bowl. When it turns into a gummy paste, add 2 tablespoons of hot water and mix again. Pour this mixture, plus 1 cup of papaya puree (per packet of gelatin puree), and _ cup of hot water into a blender. Blend for 30 seconds or so. Pour mixture into glass cups or a large bowl. Refrigerate for a couple of hours until it turns into "Jell-o" form. Enjoy!

You can also blend 1 tablespoon of minced coconut to the mixture if you want to add texture, or sprinkle it on top once you've poured the completed mixture into a bowl or cups.

Warm Raspberries and Yogurt

This is a wonderful dessert that combines and polarizes sweet and sour, warm and cold tastes. It's very delicious, and can also be used as a nourishing treat during the Undereating Phase.

Ingredients:

1 cup of fresh or frozen raspberries
1 teaspoon of honey or maple syrup
1 cup of organic, nonfat plain yogurt

Preparation:

In a small pot, add raspberries and honey (or maple syrup). Turn on the stove to a medium heat and stir. When the mixture turns fluid and begins to boil, reduce the heat and simmer for a few minutes. Take

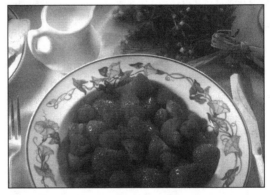

off heat and set aside for a minute. Put yogurt in a small bowl. Slowly pour the warm berries on top of the yogurt. Enjoy!

Note: You can substitute the raspberries with blueberries or blackberries. Adjust the sweetness according to your taste.

CHAPTER FOURTEEN
SEX DRIVE, POTENCY
AND ANIMAL
MAGNETISM

Thirty million men in the United States are impotent. No joke.
Richard E. Spark, M.D, Associate Clinical Professor of Medicine
at Harvard Medical School, says this number is actually an
underestimation of how many men suffer from impaired sexual
potency. Even more worrisome is the staggering percentage of
male infertility. According to the American Chemical Society,
sperm count in men worldwide is fifty percent lower than it was
fifty years ago. Needless to say, male performance is a major
problem today. The recent boom in sales of Viagra indicates just
how popular a potency drug can be in a sex-oriented society when,
ironically, such a large number of men can't perform sexually.

Sex, Power, and Instincts

Sex drive and potency were always regarded as indicators of
health and power. Since the dawn of civilization, men have
competed with each other for the best mate in order to produce the
best offspring and carry their genes into future generations. Being
unable to perform sexually or impregnate a woman was
considered a humiliating weakness. Like animal predators, human
alpha males who were leaders of their pack (group) were proud to
inseminate more women than the other males. The primal instinct
to multiply and expand territory drove males to "conquer" as
many females as possible, and the best looking among them.

According to anthropologist Desmond Morris, men used all their
senses to select a mate. There is a primal code of health and
beauty engraved in a woman's body, which attracts men.

This physical code includes visual stimulators such as a woman's curves: her breasts, hips, thighs, and butt. Ancient goddesses of fertility were depicted as all "bust and butt." A well-rounded woman was a visual indication of fertility and motherhood.

Other sensual stimulations that affected attraction, such as smell (body odor and breath) and touch (smooth skin, as opposed to dry skin) were also indicators of a woman's health. For example, having bad breath or body odor was thought to be a sign of disease, and therefore these women were considered unappealing as mates and future mothers. Women were aware of this "physical code of attractiveness" and so they would enhance their cleavage, use lotions to soften and moisturize their skin, and use perfumes and other concoctions made from herbs and flowers to improve their breath and body odor.

Men, suggested Morris, possessed their own "code of attractiveness." Females were attracted to the strongest and most dominant males. A strong man could protect and provide more for them and their children. The prime "physical" code regarding a man's appeal and level of attractiveness to women was a powerful, muscular, healthy look. Other masculine qualities, such as being aggressive enough to fight and dominate other males (leadership) were also considered powerful and attractive to women.

Male genitals were regarded as a symbol of power. Ancient weapons of war, such as spears and swords, had symbolic phallic connotations. The term "weapon" remains today a slang expression that refers to a man's penis.

The main point I'm trying to make here is that instinct has always attracted men and women to each other sexually. And further, this instinct is based on a primal code of sensual (aesthetic) attraction. I assume that this primal, instinctual code is still within us, although the rules of the game have changed. Men no longer need to be physically manly (masculine and hard) in order to be successful in life, or with women, and women don't need to be voluptuous to be considered attractive. As a matter of fact, many men today find women who have a lean and firm look to be most attractive, and many women today are attracted to men who look soft and out-of-shape.

My question is whether these changes in physical codes of attraction, in both men and women today, have had an effect on potency and fertility. I believe it has.

Modern society has created new standards for success. Thousands of years ago, it was necessary for a man and his family's survival that he be physically powerful. Possessing a combination of intelligence, masculinity, and potency was the standard of success. In biblical times, and later on, kings, rulers, and leaders were often involved in physical fights or duels. Bravery was an adored virtue and chivalry was an inherent part of a man's life.

Today, most men no longer need physical power as a means to survive, and being physically brave isn't required to succeed. Money and wealth now seem to be the most predominant parameters for power. Today, if a man has money and accumulated wealth but is not a "physical specimen," a large number of women overlook this, and are still happy to hook up. It seems as though having a "big pocket" has taken the place of having a "big phallus."

I see many men who are out-of-shape and don't seem to care about their physical appearance. They suffer from ailments such as high blood pressure, chronic constipation, and obesity, yet they continue abusing themselves with bad diets and excessive drinking. In spite of this, these men are successful in modern society because they're smart enough to make loads of money. It's my contention that the society we live in today no longer emphasizes or encourages the use of some of our most primal instincts in order to survive or thrive. I would even go further by saying that we live in an environment that emasculates men.

We do, however, still adore athletes for their physical performance and masculine, muscular look. And we also greatly admire and respect artists, scientists, and other creative types for their "creative power" and "powerful" minds. I believe it's this primal instinct which lies within us all that still attracts us to both physical and mental power, even though the emphasis and importance placed on physical prowess has so diminished.

In my opinion, the confusion about gender identity today, both sexually and aesthetically, is one reason for the rise of what I believe are artificial standards which too often take the place of natural, primal, instinctual standards. And, as I've noted earlier; when instincts are inhibited, confusion, anxiety, and poor performance result.

Male Performance Factors

Men's ability to perform sexually depends on many health-related factors that work synergistically. The most important ones are:

1. Neuro-Health: to sense psychogenic (such as visual) and physical (such as sensual, touch) stimulation for sexual arousal.
2. Hormonal Balance: to keep optimum testosterone levels in conjunction with other hormones.
3. Vascular Health: which allows an uncompromised flow of blood to the right body parts. This includes vasodilators: factors in the form of enzymes and other substances, such as NOS and cyclic GMP (cGMP) which enforce local blood flow to the genitals until a full erection occurs.
4. Mental Health: to feel sexually confident and able to handle stress and anxiety.

All of the above work together to achieve full sexual performance. If any one is not intact, impotency may result.

There's enough data today to show the correlation between impotency and chronic diseases such as diabetes, heart problems, high blood pressure, and high cholesterol. There's also a clear connection between low levels of testosterone—or high estrogen and high prolactin (the female hormone that stimulates milk production)—with male disability to perform sexually. Stress is another major factor in male performance. Psychologists and other therapists make a fortune attempting to heal and console men who have lost their sex drive or ability to perform.

Potency and Diet

When looking deeper into what causes male performance problems, I've realized that many, if not most of them, could be avoided by simply following a healthy diet and by practicing different methods of exercise that help manage stress. The connection between diet and potency is well documented and supported with clinical research. It shows a clear correlation between diet, exercise, and hormonal balance. Hormonal deficiency-related diseases affect libido, potency, and fertility.

The Pottenger Cat Study (see the following) illustrates the extreme and dramatic effects of deficient diets (diets that lack live food and enzymes) on the degradation of consequent generations of cats. Even if you're skeptical about the relevance of this study to human beings, it should at least make you wonder whether maintaining a deficient diet can affect human potency—and consequently the ability to create new, healthy generations.

The Pottenger Cat Study

The Pottenger Cat Study, conducted between 1932 and 1942, was the first clinical report dealing with the process of intergenerational degradation resulting from a deficient diet.

The study used approximately nine hundred cats, divided into two control groups. One control group of cats was fed a raw food diet including raw meat, raw milk, and cod liver oil. The other control group was put on a deficient diet. The health of the first, second, third, and fourth generation of all cats was studied, with a focus on their immunity, potency, and fertility.

The results were stunning. Those cats on the deficient diets could not produce a fourth generation, and the first generation already showed the first signs of degradation, such as heart problems, underactive thyroid and bladder, arthritis, inflammation of the nervous system, and various infections. Second and third generations of cats on the deficient diet also suffered from an acceleration of these symptoms and showed a general decrease in the health of reproductive organs. Males showed a failure in active general decrease in the health of reproductive organs. Males showed a failure in active spermatogenesis (meaning they had low sperm count and weak sperm). Miscarriages accounted for up to seventy percent in second-generation deficient cats. Skin allergies were frequent and got worse with each subsequent generation. The third generation cats were so deficient that none survived beyond the sixth month. Needless to say, there was no fourth generation of deficient cats.

In contrast, those cats that were given raw food ("normal cats") were healthy in all generations. Their internal organs were fully developed, and the immune systems of all four generations of these cats were fully intact, with no signs of infections or allergies. They reproduced one homogeneous generation after another, all in good health.

It's interesting to note that when the second generation of "deficient cats" was put back on a raw food diet, some of the deficiency-related symptoms, such as allergies, diminished and by the fourth generation some cats had fully restored immune systems.

There also seemed to be a general connection between hypothyroidism (low thyroid) and male sterility. Eighty-three percent of male "deficient" cats in the second generation were sterile. Fifty-three percent of second-generation female "deficient" cats showed under-developed ovaries.

According to a Kellogg Report by Joseph Beasley, M.D. and Jerry Swift, M.A., forty-four percent of thirty million couples surveyed in the United States in 1980 with a woman of childbearing age were unable to have children. In 1965, there were 482,000 couples with a wife younger than thirty who were classified as infertile. By 1976, the number of infertile couples rose to 920,000. Among black couples (ages twenty to twenty-four), the proportion of infertile couples went up from three percent to fifteen percent in the eleven-year span from 1965–1976.

Dr. Pottenger theorized that there are similarities between malformations found in animals and those found in humans.

My points here are that:

1. *I firmly believe there is indeed a direct connection between diet, health, sexual performance, and fertility for both men and women.*

2. *The lack of raw foods, live nutrients, and enzymes in the typical American diet makes it a deficient diet, which causes unpleasant symptoms as well as health maladies.*

I believe, furthermore, that the Pottenger Cat Study throws significant light on what may be contributing to the acceleration of immunodeficiency and chronic diseases in our culture, such as cancer, hypothyroidism, sterility, hyperactivity, and depression.

The Syndrome of Taking Drugs

As noted, chronic diseases such as heart disease (arteriosclerosis), high blood pressure, high cholesterol, as well as depression, can cause impotency. Blood pressure medications, such as beta antagonists, heart medications such as alpha antagonists, and some anti-depression drugs, can also cause impotency as a side effect. So, here's the catch: in order to solve one problem people take drugs, but drugs can create other problems. Disease-related impotence is more often than not treated with drugs that, ironically, may badly affect sexual performance.

When you hear about miracle pills, just remember that in spite of a low statistical rate of side effects, most popular potency pills don't work for everyone. And those suspected to experience side effects are more likely to be those who need it most. As just stated, men who take blood pressure medications or who suffer from heart problems and take medication often suffer from impotency. Then, when tempted to try a potency drug to restore their virility, side effects as severe as coma or death can occur.

I'm not against the use of drugs per se. Taking the right medication can improve or save your life. I'd like to strongly suggest here that if you suffer from male performance-related problems, go and seek out professional help. I also recommend that you ask your doctor and pharmacist about the side effects of all drugs prescribed to you, so at least you're aware.

Potency—Natural Methods to Enhance Potency

As noted, there are many factors involved in men's sexual function. There isn't enough space here to discuss the entire scientific complex of hormonal, neurological, and glandular factors, which are essential for proper male performance. To put things simply, let me just say that hormonal balance is a key to men's sexual function. If one hormone, such as adrenaline, is overactive or if another hormone such as the thyroid is underactive, impotency may occur.

The hormone responsible for sex drive (in both men and women) is testosterone. This male hormone is responsible for some critical functions, such as:

- Development of male sex organs
- Regulating healthy sperm production
- Activation and maintenance of sex drive for both men and women
- Maintenance of strong bones
- Build muscles and burn fat for both men and women

What Affects Testosterone Production, Sex Drive and Libido

When testosterone levels decline, sex drive and libido diminishes. There are many reasons for inadequate testosterone production. Some of them are related to disease and others to lifestyle stressors, diet, and aging.

I'd like to discuss the most common things that affect testosterone production, and therefore sex drive and libido. As noted, there is a connection between diet and potency; and bad diets can negatively affect testosterone levels in the blood. Chronic low-calorie and crash diets, mineral deficiencies of zinc, magnesium, copper, or iodine, protein, or essential fatty acid deficiencies, all may cause low testosterone production in the short or long run. To make matters worse, crash diets or anorexic diets can badly affect normal thyroid production. Having a low thyroid may cause high prolactin (the lactating hormone). High prolactin levels block the production of testosterone as well as the growth hormone. High prolactin may cause breast enlargement and feminization in men.

The market is saturated with over-the-counter supplements to boost the thyroid, and prescription thyroid hormones are in widespread use. The thyroid hormones regulate metabolism.

Those who take thyroid supplements to boost their thyroid in order to lose weight often don't realize that having an overactive thyroid is as dangerous as having an underactive thyroid. When the level of thyroid hormones is too high in the blood, it creates a situation in which more testosterone is converted to estrogen (the female hormone), and this brings side effects with it, including the feminization of men's bodies and a declining sex drive.

Stress is also a major factor in healthy testosterone production. Excessive physical or mental stress may cause a direct diminution in testosterone production as well as lagging libido.

Aging is another factor that affects testosterone. The more you age, the less testosterone is produced in your body.

Considering all the above, a healthy diet that supplies all essential nutrients, and therefore energy, as well as stress management methods, such as relaxation techniques, regular exercise, and a proper nutritional program that helps slow the aging process, are all natural methods that work as a first defense against low testosterone. I truly believe that the best way to keep your vigor high is to follow a cycle of daily detoxification, and then consume nutritional meals that make you feel satisfied, compensated, and relaxed every night.

Overtraining Vs. Your Sex Drive

Overtraining may rob you of your testosterone. Avoid overstressing your body with long, obsessive, daily, physical training routines. It's critical to take at least one-to-two days off per week. Rest is part of the training cycle and is necessary for recuperation and strength gain.

Symptoms related to overtraining, such as hypothyroidism (low thyroid), a sluggish metabolism, muscle tightening and cramping, exhaustion, depression, and sleep disorders, may also occur or be exacerbated by a deficient diet. Low-calorie diets, crash diets, low protein diets, raw food deficient diets, as well as diets deficient in essential nutrients (such as vitamins, minerals and essential fatty acids), may not satisfy your body's need to recuperate fully from intense physical strain. Any exercise routine combined with malnutrition may lead to overtraining-related symptoms.

Aphrodisiac Supplements (that enhance libido)

The word aphrodisiac is attached to many herbs, potions, lotions, and nutritional formulas. Unfortunately most aphrodisiac supplements don't work. Commercial companies try to cash in on this or that exotic herb, promising great results, but the truth is that it's very unlikely one single herb can help restore healthy performance in those who suffer from impotency. There are many factors that are critical for sexual performance. Isolating and targeting one or another usually isn't good enough. Many people who experience diminished libido and impaired performance suffer due to a complex set of factors (such as neurological, glandular, hormonal and mental factors), which have taken them out of balance. Often, both physical and psychological issues are involved in impaired sexual performance.

The Warrior Diet–
Instinctual Living and Potency

As I've said before, the Warrior Diet isn't a cure for everything. Nevertheless, it encourages instinctual living and thus unleashes the power of your instincts. Primal instincts are based on an inner wisdom of your body to react spontaneously, to both physical and psychological stimulations. An instinct, once triggered, should activate all factors necessary for its specific action. Conversely, when instincts aren't intact or can't be activated, the body cannot coordinate the different factors necessary for healthy performance. This is exactly when problems occur. Isolating one factor or another as the culprit for impotence is a popular method used by many doctors, who often prescribe specific drugs to treat specific problems.

Nevertheless, I believe that the revival of sexual instincts is the most natural and powerful way to restore and enhance potency. Once you unleash the power of your instincts you'll be able to perform spontaneously simply by letting your own body's wisdom follow through with the right action. The notion that you can increase your vigor and improve your performance by improving your diet, exercising regularly, and living instinctually may sound simplistic and romantic, especially in these times when drugs and synthetic supplements are the basis of most popular quick-fix methods. Regardless, those who experience the power of raw living know what I'm talking about.

Craving Aphrodisiac Foods Instinctively

On a related matter, I truly believe we often instinctively crave foods that enhance sexuality. These aphrodisiac foods aren't always mysterious, esoteric, or exotic. Actually, you likely consume some very powerful aphrodisiac foods and herbs quite often. Meat, nuts, seeds, seafood, and wine are all considered to contain some sex-enhancing properties. Herbs and spices such as ginseng and gingko, cinnamon and vanilla beans, have been used for thousands of years as natural aids or remedies to enhance sexual performance.

Meat and seafood are abundant in zinc, as well as other essential minerals. Maintaining optimum mineral levels is critical for optimum hormonal balance. Zinc is necessary for testosterone production, male virility, and sperm production. Red meat is high in the amino acid arginine. Arginine is essential for the production of nitric oxide (NO)—a neuro-substance necessary for erections. Ginseng and gingko are herbs that stimulate the production of nitric oxide through the enzyme nitric oxide synthase (NOS). Gingko optimizes blood circulation in the brain and ginseng is believed to be an adaptogenic herb that helps the body handle stress. These qualities make these herbs potent aphrodisiacs.

There are other aphrodisiac foods that traditionally were considered natural aids for sexual performance. Almonds, for instance, have been regarded as an aphrodisiac food since biblical times. The Romans thought of the almond as a symbol of men's genitals. I often recommend that people try "almond and veggie" meals for a couple of days. (For more on almonds, see the "Overeating" chapter). Almonds are naturally high in zinc, copper, and manganese. In its raw state, this nut is a mild alkalizer. I think almonds are one of the most powerful aphrodisiac foods, especially for men.

Wine has been considered an aphrodisiac for thousands of years. Taste, color, smell, and aroma are all factors that contribute to the sexual nature of this ancient nectar. A glass or two of wine has a relaxing effect, sheds inhibitions, and, from this perspective alone, is an aphrodisiac. Wine is often served as part of a romantic dinner. However, excessive drinking may work in the opposite way. Alcohol has a diminishing effect on blood testosterone and sperm count. Many guys know that when they drink too much, it reduces desire and can make them fall asleep instead of making love.

There are also some so-called exotic foods that are thought to be aphrodisiac, such as cherries, passion fruit, fertile eggs, oysters, and, of course, chocolate. All the above may or may not enhance sexual performance. Nevertheless, the placebo effect is real. If you believe a certain food is aphrodisiac, then for you it most probably is. It's not imperative to know the science behind everything you crave. Use your instincts. Whatever works for you is good, and vice versa.

As a last note for this matter, let me just mention that any food or beverage that stimulates dopamine in your brain could be a natural aid in enhancing sexual desire and performance. Coffee, tea, and hot chocolate (cocoa) are but a few examples of beverages that fall in this category.

Food and sex have been bound together for a long time. I guess this is due to the intimate connection between the two most powerful instincts that predominate in life: the instinct to survive and the instinct to multiply. Nourishment and sex give us a great sense of pleasure. Having the wisdom to satisfy both desires—for food and sex—is the art of living well. I truly believe that this wisdom lies within us all.

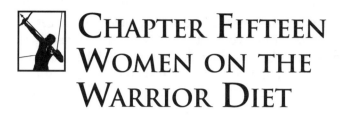

CHAPTER FIFTEEN
WOMEN ON THE
WARRIOR DIET

In spite of all the masculine connotations and machismo surrounding the Warrior Diet, I truly believe it can work equally well for women. I know women who follow my diet with great results.

Women have some specific desires and needs, such as looking healthy and attractive, losing weight, and slowing the aging process, and they are all addressed extensively in this book.

Women also need to feel a sense of freedom, to live instinctually, and especially to enjoy the satisfaction of so-called "wild" pleasures—which, unfortunately, are too often repressed or inhibited.

Artificial aesthetic standards set by Madison Avenue, and society for that matter, tend to dictate that women restrict themselves and endure the tyranny of over-restrictive dietary rules just to stay in shape. Many books on the market today attempt to capitalize on this with quick-fix fad diets built on restraint—be it calorie-counting, fat or carbohydrate restriction, or the quite popular liquid diets, based on the principle of substituting real food with allegedly "healthy" shakes.

As a result, many women today have developed a "fear" of food. Fat phobias, carbohydrate phobias, and calorie counting are all modern symptoms of weight-loss despair. Food phobias are both obsessive and dangerous, and start at an alarmingly young age. More girls suffer from anorexia and other eating disorders than ever before. Girls, as well as grown women, have fallen victim to popular culture image-makers and so-called "ideals."

Those who try fad diets often lose weight initially, but then gain it back again—and many even put on more weight. Something must be wrong here. I believe the core of the problem is the fact that, as stated above, many women today deprive themselves, which is extremely difficult to do in the long run, and their natural instincts are crushed. Following artificial body image and lifestyle standards eliminates your freedom of choice—and without feeling free you can't follow your instincts.

The Warrior Diet unleashes the power of your own instincts. If you practice it, I believe you'll naturally shed obsessive restrictions and rules while still addressing your basic needs, such as losing weight, eliminating stubborn fat, maintaining healthy skin, nails, and hair, slowing the aging process, and maybe most importantly, feeling a true sense of freedom and well-being.

Detoxification

Those people who follow the Warrior Diet will find that daily detoxification during the Undereating Phase is the best natural method for rejuvenating all body tissues. Loading up with live nutrients such as enzymes, minerals, vitamins, and flavones, which come from live veggies and fruits, cleanse your body and protect you from environmental and internal toxins. There's enough research today that shows the correlation between live nutrients—such as carotene complex—with fertility, healthy skin, and immunity. Loading your body with live enzymes is vital to slowing the aging process. Enzymes, such as lipase, also play an essential role in fat loss.

Overeating

All diets today tell you not to overeat. However, as I say throughout this book, overeating, when done the right way, can work for you. Many women binge at night and feel guilty afterwards. I explain in the "Overeating Phase" chapter that bingeing isn't bad if you know how and when to do it. *Nighttime* is the right time to overeat.

This said, the Warrior Diet definitely does not advocate uncontrolled compulsive bingeing—quite the opposite. When you practice overeating, you should be in full control.

Overeating is a relative matter. For some it means consuming a 500-calorie meal, and for others it means consuming a 1,500-calorie meal. If you follow the Warrior Diet rules of eating, you'll know instinctively what, when, and how much to eat, and when to stop. You'll learn how to trust your feminine instinct. If nothing else, this will give you a tremendous sense of freedom, something other diets don't offer. Moreover, following the Warrior Diet should accelerate your metabolism and therefore should, in time, allow you to eat more.

Hormonal Fluctuations

Women often suffer from hormonal fluctuations. There's substantial data that shows the link between diet, nutrition, and the hormonal system. Unbalanced diets often cause nutrient deficiencies or excessive toxicity. When this happens, women often suffer from severe symptoms of hormonal fluctuations, such as weight gain, mood swings, bloating, water retention, headaches, nausea, and hot flashes. Conversely, following a diet that *detoxifies* your body while *nourishing* it with all essential nutrients may help alleviate these symptoms.

On a related matter, women who take hormonal replacements should be aware of the dangers and side effects of this therapy. I'm not against or in favor of hormonal therapy; I believe this decision should be left to you and your physician. Nevertheless, the Warrior Diet can be of great benefit for those that do undergo such treatment. By practicing daily detoxification, and with the right supplementation, you can help your liver detoxify or neutralize hormone derivatives, such as estrogenic substances, and thus reduce the risk of hormone-related side effects.

Stubborn Fat

Many women suffer from stubborn fat-related problems. Stubborn fat is a major issue, which most diets don't address. Those who have stubborn fat (usually around the thighs, butt, and hips) should find the Warrior Diet—and the suggested nutritional supplements—helpful in fighting and eliminating it. For more on stubborn fat, see Chapter 7.

To quickly sum up, the Warrior Diet is an instinctual diet that allows *everyone* to feel the power of raw living—to experience a real sense of freedom and at the same time enjoy the pleasure of reaching full satisfaction from meals—while having the gratification of increased energy and an improved physical appearance. So don't let my references to ancient warriors dissuade you from trying the Warrior Diet. As stated right at the beginning, when I refer to the term "warrior" it is to an instinct that is deep within us all —both women and men—that can be triggered by practicing this diet.

Unlike many popular diet books, we have chosen not to fill *The Warrior Diet* with stories of personal success, male or female. However, some women may wish to hear how the diet works from a woman's point of view. For these women, I am including Diana Holtzberg's own story.

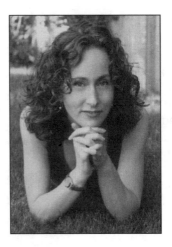

Diana Holtzberg's Experience with the Warrior Diet

Out of nowhere, at the age of 30, I suddenly developed severe allergies. Mystified, I went to a traditional allergist and tested positive to "almost everything." He prescribed three drugs and a few years of regular desensitization shots. But the drugs made me feel worse and I wasn't keen to have all those shots.

There had to be a better way. I found a holistic internist—who quickly laid the blame on a combination of my poor eating habits and history of antibiotic use. Frankly, I was shocked. Until then, I had no clue that there might be a relationship between my diet and current predicament. He also determined I had a mild case of EBV (Chronic Fatigue Syndrome) and Candida Albicans.

As a kid, my breakfasts were sugar-saturated bowls of cereal, interspersed with weekend brunches of bacon and eggs, bagels with cream cheese, and smoked fishes. A typical lunch was a canned meat dish and cookies, washed down with a pop. Dinner was usually "meat and potatoes", or a frozen TV Dinner, followed by sweets.

My adult diet was more of the same: a bagel with cream cheese for breakfast, and a sandwich, with chips, and cookies was a typical lunch. I had a candy bar every afternoon when I was crashing, and evenings weren't complete without a brownie, a piece of cake, or cookies.

On this doctor's advice, I modified my diet and lifestyle, gave up refined sugars, a large majority of the overly-processed foods I'd so loved, ate way more vegetables, began to purchase organic products, and didn't drink any alcohol for a couple of years. Yet, with all these changes, I still didn't feel as energetic, clear-headed, or as healthy as I hoped to. In fact, I still felt tired much of the time.

After years of trying different practitioners and healing methods, which left me in no better condition, I finally decided to try the Warrior Diet. It wasn't until I began to practice this diet almost two years ago that I really started to feel and see major signs of improvement.

The Warrior Diet has greatly enhanced my life. I have much more energy now, and my body is leaner, better defined, and stronger. My allergies have diminished and my Candida is history.

What I love about this diet is that I can experiment and customize it, and I never feel deprived. Food is one of my great passions, and now that I've developed a subtle palate, I adore the taste of whole foods. I have a huge appetite these days, but remain thin and in good shape.

Given my personal experience, I can strongly recommend the Warrior Diet to any woman disenchanted by her past dietary failures—and eager to embrace a life of renewed energy, well being and enhanced physical appearance. I'm thrilled to be helping bring Ori's message to a larger audience.

CHAPTER SIXTEEN
THE WARRIOR DIET
NUTRITIONAL
SUPPLEMENTS

I originally created the Warrior Diet Nutritional Supplements for my personal use since I didn't trust the quality or integrity of most commercial protein powders and natural supplements (such as probiotics and enzymes) that are on the market today. I decided to produce them myself to ensure that the quality wasn't compromised.

Many popular diets today, conversely, are built on the principal of consuming meal replacements instead of eating real, whole food. What makes these plans even worse is the fact that a large number of commercial meal replacements are loaded with food additives and chemicals. As hunter-predators we all need to eat real food. Any diet program that tells you otherwise is misleading. This said, nutritional supplements may be of great benefit if they are taken to enhance the nutritional composition of your meals, not as a substitute for them.

I take the Warrior Diet Nutritional Supplements on a daily basis. Most of them are derived from whole foods, and should be eaten like food. The main idea behind these supplements is to enrich the nutritive composition of your diet, especially when certain foods or live nutrients aren't available. Most of these supplements have been designed to support you during the Undereating Phase. As noted, they give you easy access to high-quality nutritional products, such as protein powders, minerals, enzymes, probiotics, and greens, which may be helpful to detoxify and nourish your mind and body during this phase, as well as before and after your workout.

Production of the Warrior Diet Nutritional Supplements

It took me years to improve upon and finally produce the line of Warrior Diet supplements. During this time I discovered that homemade products are one thing, and manufacturing them for widespread use is quite another. While my friends and I have enjoyed some of them (such as Warrior Growth Serum and Warrior Milk) for a while, what seemed great when homemade became, at times, something completely different on the production line. I wasn't ready to compromise.

It's difficult to describe just how excited and surprised my friends were when they tried these homemade nutritional supplements. They said the protein powders tasted so good they felt like bingeing on them. It remains my goal to create alternative nutritional products that are as good as homemade products, and even better.

I searched for what seemed an eternity for someone I could trust who could help me produce this line. After many disappointments and delays, the right person finally approached me while I was writing this book. When I first met Dr. Robert J. Marshall, Ph.D., CCN, he was excited by the project, and I soon realized that we shared similar ideas. Dr. Marshall has outstanding credentials. He holds degrees from the University of Dayton and Purdue University. He is an internationally trained biochemist and certified clinical nutritionist, and was the President of the International and American Association of Clinical Nutritionists. He is a member of the American Society of Tropical Medicine and Hygiene, and is currently the Clinic Director of a well-known chronic disease treatment facility, which he has managed for almost thirty years. Dr. Marshall is famous for his uncompromising integrity, and I'm pleased that he is overseeing quality control as well as helping me produce the Warrior Diet supplements.

Product Safety

As a final note for this introduction, I'd like to address the issue of safety. Many people are concerned today about bovine dairy products, primarily as a result of the widely reported Hoof-and-Mouth disease and Mad Cow disease. Others are troubled about the chemicals and hormones often found in dairy products. I'm aware of these concerns and have taken them seriously into account. The Warrior Diet Nutritional Supplements are made from clean, chemical and drug-free, undenatured food sources, including the protein powders. Our air-dried colostrum and whey are derived from the milk of healthy cows, which are treated humanely and fed grain and grass that are free of chemically based pesticides, with absolutely no animal by-products added to any feed. As a standard safety measure, all final products are lab-tested for chemical, metal, viral, and bacterial contents. Safety and quality control are top priorities for all Warrior Diet supplements. As mentioned, I take them on a daily basis.

The Supplements

1. Warrior Growth Serum

Warrior Growth Serum is a proprietary blend of undenatured air-dried colostrum produced from organically fed, drug-free, healthy cows, with other nutrients, such as grade A inulin and CLA, which support the metabolic system. This powder is high in immunosupportive protein, growth factors, and lactoferin—ingredients often missing in other dairy protein powders. The colostrum is derived from the first milking of a lactating cow.

As far as I know, Warrior Growth Serum is the most potent protein powder available today. In its raw state, this protein powder tastes so delicious that some friends who've tried it actually said they felt like bingeing on it. Warrior Growth Serum is sweetened with grade A inulin (FOS), which is an extremely low-calorie, low glycemic, oligosacaride natural sweetener that's derived from chicory.

According to Dr. Marshall, Warrior Growth Serum can actually induce a five-fold increase in good bacteria in the large intestine in just four weeks of use. In addition to its pleasant, sweet taste, FOS helps feed the friendly bacteria in the digestive tract and, therefore, works as an aid for better digestion and assimilation.

I like to chew the powder in its raw state, but you can also mix it with water and have it as a creamy shake. Warrior Growth Serum is best taken on an empty stomach during the Undereating Phase, or before or after your workout. It can also be mixed with other protein shakes to enhance their potency, or sprinkled on top of fish, eggs, or carb meals to maximize their nutritional composition.

- **Those people concerned about Mad Cow disease, and its effect on bovine products, should know that the Warrior Diet dairy proteins are derived and produced from healthy cows that are not fed animal feeds or grains with chemically based pesticides, and the final products are checked carefully for impurities.**

2. Warrior Milk

Warrior Milk is a proprietary blend of specially processed, pesticide-free whey isolate, with growth serum and other nutrients that enhance its potency and assimilation. Warrior Milk is a new hybrid of super-protein powder, which as far as I am aware, goes above and beyond any protein powder or meal replacement available today. It's high in immuno-supportive protein and growth factors, as well as lactoferin. This protein powder can be used as a substitute for a cooked protein meal at times these foods aren't available. It tastes delicious, and is best taken right after your workout.

Warrior Milk should help you satisfy your daily protein requirement. Due to its protein composition, Warrior Milk is a great supplemental food for those interested in accelerating the anabolic process of building muscles. Warrior Milk is partly sweetened with FOS, a grade A extremely low-calorie natural sweetener derived from chicory.

3. Warrior Greens

Warrior Greens is a proprietary blend of low-temperature air-dried, organically grown greens. It's made from a special combination of green raw grass with wild-grown blue-green algae, grade A Japanese chlorella, and grade 10 Noni from India. Warrior Greens are processed in a way that preserves all life forces within the product—including vitamins, minerals, food enzymes, chlorophyll, flavones, and all vital nutrients, which are essential for detoxification, digestion, and overall health. Warrior Greens are best taken on an empty stomach during the Undereating Phase. This supplement gives you easy access to a very potent live grass.

You can also sprinkle it on top of your food, whether protein or carbs, to improve the composition of your meal and enhance nutrient assimilation. Warrior Greens is a wonderful alkalizer, and is naturally a most potent aid to combat environmental and radioactive toxins.

4. Warrior Probiotics

Warrior Probiotics is, in my opinion, the most potent blend of live, friendly bacteria, essential for the integrity of your gastrointestinal tract flora. Friendly bacteria help protect the body from bacterial and viral infections. They secrete antibiotic substances, which work as a natural aid in destroying pathogenic (harmful) bacteria as well as yeast and parasites. Probiotics are necessary for digestion and elimination of toxins. They also help in the production of certain B vitamins, and antioxidant enzymes, such as SOD and glutathione. Without the right balance of probiotics in the system, digestion and elimination are compromised. Probiotics protect the body from allergens and detoxify the colon from undigested protein and toxins.

I believe Warrior Probiotics are a step ahead of other probiotic supplements. They're made from live soil bacteria, including the largest variety of natural, organic, friendly bacteria. In the past, people ingested these bacteria through food. Today the soil has been greatly depleted of these friendly bacteria, which is probably one reason why so many people today suffer from digestive problems, yeast infections, bloating, allergies, and constipation. Warrior Probiotics re-introduce these soil bacteria to your body. I can't emphasize enough the importance of probiotics to your health and vitality. Warrior Probiotics is the best supplement I know of to ensure maximum protein utilization, proper digestion, and elimination.

Note:

Athletes and bodybuilders who consume large amounts of protein should be especially concerned about protein utilization and the danger of undigested toxins in the colon.

Warrior Enzymes

5. Warrior-zyme

Warrior-zyme is a proprietary blend of live enzymes with high protease and lipase enzymes. Loading your body with live enzymes is believed to be a natural way to help keep a youthful appearance. Enzymes, such as protease, work systemically as an antioxidant, anti-inflammatory, antiallergenic, and anticancerous agent. Other enzymes, such as lipase, help regulate proper fat metabolism and the breakdown of fat into energy. Lipase is believed to have antiaging properties.

Live enzymes help the digestion and elimination of food. Eating cooked and processed food, solely, leaves many people with large enzyme deficits. Enzyme deficiencies may contribute to a variety of problems, such as indigestion, constipation, allergies, fatigue, mood swings, PMS, and skin rashes. Loading your body with live enzymes could be the first defense against enzyme deficiency-related problems.

Warrior (living plant) Enzymes are made using a breakthrough proprietary fermentation process that starts with various forms of aspergillus, and yields highly purified, fully active enzymes free of toxic residues, thereby helping eliminate the risk of immune system compromise.

Enzymes sold on the market today vary widely in quality. If an enzyme originates from an animal source, its potency may vary a great deal, and its toxic tag-along (such as pesticides and hormones) is a fact of life. On the other hand, if the enzymes are made from fungi, they may be free of pesticides, insecticides, and other toxins, but almost always contain remnant fungi, like aspergillus, which can be immune-compromising. Warrior-zyme, which is rich in living plant enzymes, delivers the most potent and purest source of these enzymes. Experience the difference for yourself. The enzyme activity of Warrior-zyme is based on food chemical code (FCC) units, which are recognized by the FDA. These enzymes are derived from aspergillus, a fungal plant source. After production, these enzymes are highly purified, so there is no remaining aspergillus. Warrior-zyme is a cut above, not only in enzyme activity, but, of equal importance, in purity.

Warrior-zyme is high-potency enzyme power to help your digestion and detoxification. It contains protease, lipase, amylase, cellulase, invertase, lactase, and maltase to help digest protein, fat, starch, sugars, and fiber. These enzymes are in a base of organic apple-cider vinegar powder, which delivers an organic acid-rich substrate to enhance the body's own enzyme synthesis. Warrior-zyme is made from once-living sources using a breakthrough proprietary fermentation process starting with aspergillus, and yielding the most highly purified fully active enzymes, free of any toxic aspergillus residues.

Each 500 mg vegetable capsule of Warrior-zyme provides:

Protease	30,000 HUT (Hemoglobin Unit Tyrosine base)
Lipase	145 LU (Lipase Unit)
Amylase	10,000 DU (Alpha-amylase Dextrinizing Units)
Cellulase	600 CU (Cellulase Unit)
Invertase	0.75 IAU (Invertase Activity Unit)
Lactase	360 LacU (Lactase Unit)
Maltase	250 DP (Degrees of Diastatic Power)

60 capsules per bottle. 100% pure vegetable capsules in a base of organic apple cider vinegar powder, (33% acetobacter), with no toxic binders, fillers, or flowing agents.

6. Warrior Male Performance Support

I created this formula a few years ago to help a man who, at that time, suffered from age-related problems that affected his sexual performance. The result was astonishing. He said that my formula made him feel young and vigorous, something he hadn't felt for a long time.

Others who've tried Warrior Male Performance Support have said it dramatically enhanced their physical performance, mental sharpness, and sexual potency.

Male performance can be affected by various factors, such as an unhealthy lifestyle, stress, or age. The Warrior Male Performance Support formula is a proprietary blend of nutrients and herbs that naturally mimics the way testosterone works in your body. It also helps regulate certain hormones and neurotransmitters in the brain to enhance natural synergy between body and mind. This is, I believe, the only complete nutritional option for consumers.

It enhances male performance through three essential factors:

1. Testosterone Precursors—to enhance and accelerate testosterone production and synthesis.
2. Vasodilators—to help ensure ample flow of blood and oxygen to every important part of the body.
3. Cerebral supporters—to maintain healthy nerve impulses and hormonal balance in the brain.

In addition, it contains antioxidants, herbs, vitamins, proteins, and minerals to keep the mind and body naturally energized, support prostate health, and optimize sexual potency. Unlike illicit steroids, or even Viagra, this is an all-natural drug-free product. There are many natural supplements on the market that claim to boost potency. As far as I know, none of them really work. Yet greedy marketing wizards are pushing these cheap formulas. The people behind these products often know they don't work; nevertheless, they make millions through ads and infomercials based on a one-time sale. If you've ever tried these supplements, you probably know what I'm talking about.

The Warrior Male Performance Support supplement is not what you've seen or tried before. So far, the response to this supplement has been so outstanding, it sounds almost miraculous. Nevertheless, let me note here again that by following the Warrior Diet you'll naturally energize your mind and body. This alone warrants healthy performance. Some people like to take this supplement before and after exercise to accelerate the anabolic effect of the workout. Others like to take it simply because it "picks them up" sexually.

If you'd like more information about this product, please call toll free: **866-WAR DIET (927-3438).**

7. Warrior Stubborn Fat Burner

The Warrior Stubborn Fat Burner is a proprietary blend of nutrients, designed to help maintain a healthy, lean body. It works naturally to help alleviate stubborn fat-related problems through three essential factors:

1. Estrogen Blockers — a potent combination of flavonoids and herbs that occupy estrogen receptors and thus protect the body from estrogen-related symptoms.
2. Anti-aromatasing — It supports your body's anti-aromatasing actions, and thus helps support normal testosterone levels and healthy hormonal balance.
3. Alpha 2 Antagonist — It may help regulate and activate certain adrenal receptors in fat tissues, thus, accelerating fat burning.

In addition, it contains antioxidant nutrients, herbs, and flavonoids that support healthy metabolism and help detoxify the liver.

If you want to learn more about how to deal with stubborn fat-related problems, see Chapter 7. Allow me to repeat myself by saying that following a healthy diet and keeping a steady exercise routine is vital for keeping lean. Supplements can only help accelerate the results.

Warrior Live Minerals—
Highly Ionized Coral Minerals:

Mineral supplementation is a top priority of the Warrior Diet. Minerals are the building blocks for all body tissues. Besides playing a critical role in all enzymatic and hormonal actions, minerals are essential for balancing the pH in your system. There's enough research that shows the correlation between having an overly acidic body and chronic diseases such as arthritis and cancer. The body optimally needs a pH that is slightly alkaline in order to function properly. An acidic pH creates a hostile internal environment, making the body struggle to get the nutrients it needs to maintain optimal health. The more acidic you become, the worse you feel. As the body pH comes into better balance, your body easily assimilates minerals, as well as other nutrients, that were difficult to absorb at a lower, more acidic pH. Keeping your body in the proper alkaline pH range is one of the most important things you can do for yourself.

The Warrior Minerals are derived from a once-living coral source. Coral Minerals are highly ionized and contain the optimum ratio of calcium, magnesium, zinc, copper, and manganese, and other trace minerals. The ionic form of the Warrior Minerals is the most biologically active form, and the most absorbable.

Calcium is the #1 mineral by quantity in the human body. It's biochemically necessary to life, and a secret of your youth. The human body may commonly become depleted of soft tissue calcium reserves over time. Calcium plays a key role in neutralizing acidic compounds (usually toxins) anywhere in the body before damage takes place. After they're neutralized, the body can then easily excrete these acidic compounds. Otherwise, they begin to accumulate in the body—first in the joints and later in the organs and glands, choking off life. Ionized calcium is critical for cleansing.

The Warrior Ionized Minerals are easy to absorb. Many forms of calcium are very difficult to assimilate. You can be deficient in calcium even if large amounts are present in your diet. Calcium typically requires a healthy amount of stomach acid (hydrochloric acid) to break it down into a bioavailable, ionized form. Many people do not produce enough stomach acid and therefore suffer from calcium deficiencies, as well as other mineral deficiencies. Aging, stress, and disease are all factors that cause a decline in stomach-acid production. The calcium in Warrior Minerals is a unique ionized form. This means that stomach acid isn't required to absorb it.

Otto Heinrich Warburg won the Nobel Prize in 1931 for proving that cancer cells thrive in anaerobic (oxygen-free) environments. An overacidic body is one way to create a low-oxygen environment. Researchers in the 1940s and 1950s noticed that people with cancer, arthritis, and other degenerative diseases all suffered from calcium deficiencies. Researchers know that cancer cannot survive in an alkaline environment. Ionized calcium is the key mineral to keep your pH closer to ideal.

First Defense

Warrior Minerals are free of toxic metals, which are found in many colloidal mineral products on the market today. Warrior Coral Minerals contain 24 percent calcium, 12 percent magnesium, with the balance being trace minerals. It even contains trace minerals such as praseodymium and yttrium, found only in highly fertile soil. The optimum ratio of macrominerals, such as calcium and magnesium, to trace minerals is the key to mineral body-rebuilding properties. As noted, Warrior Live Minerals may be the first defense against radiation. The chelation properties of minerals and the alkalizing factor protect the body from radioactive toxins (both environmental and internal) while enhancing the immune system for optimum health.

Active men can deplete their bodies of minerals in a matter of hours. Long, intense exercise increases lactic acid in the body. Proper mineral supplementation helps protect the body from mineral deficiencies, and alkalize the system to optimum levels, thus increasing endurance and accelerating recovery.

Proper mineral supplementation prevents mineral deficiencies. Ionized minerals help optimize the acid-base balance in your body. A healthy pH warrants healthy metabolism and overall health.

Master Your pH Balance

Active men and women who are engaged in intense exercise routines, as well as those who suffer from overacidity may need to ingest a large amount of live ionized minerals in order to obtain the desired alkaline effect. The solution is to combine these three supplements, which work together synergistically to master your pH balance.

8. Warrior Live Minerals (capsules)

Warrior Live Mineral capsules is a unique coral mineral powder, rich in ionic calcium, magnesium, and trace minerals. It is fortified with vitamin D3 (the active form of vitamin D, which is essential for calcium absorption).

9. Warrior Live Minerals (powder)

Warrior Live Minerals is a unique coral powder, rich in ionic calcium, magnesium, and trace minerals (not colloidal minerals). Coral minerals have spectacular tissue bioavailability when mixed with Warrior Live Aloe Powder, which has been strongly fortified with negative ions. Warrior Live Aloe Powder offers ultra high energy potential when mixed with the Live Coral Minerals. Most people can feel a burst of energy within a few minutes after drinking (or chewing) this dynamic duo powder.

10. Warrior Live Aloe Powder

This highly charged, concentrated organic aloe powder is combined with pure organic pomegranate, a natural chelating agent that bonds the minerals to the aloe's amino acids, thereby targeting them to the organs and endocrine glands.

11. Warrior Premier
Norwegian Cod Liver Oil (capsules)

Rich in a most potent natural biological form of vitamin D, cod liver oil is an absolute requirement for absorbing calcium. Warrior Premier Norwegian Cod Liver Oil is the best quality U.S.P. grade oil (not animal feed grade). Those who aren't exposed to sunlight or spend most of their time indoors may need to supplement their body with Warrior Norwegian Cod Liver Oil to help keep optimum levels of active vitamin D.

Future Products—to come:

- **Warrior Colostrum Bar**
- **Warrior Supper Meal Bar**
- **Warrior Protein Bar**
- **Warrior Glutamine Chewables**

We're in the process of developing more new products. All are unique to the Warrior Diet. For more information on current or future products, please call toll free: 866-WAR DIET (927-3438).

Your input and opinions are important to us. If you'd like to comment on the supplements, please email them to: **www.warriordiet.org**

ABOUT THE AUTHOR

Ori Hofmekler is a modern Renaissance man whose life has been driven by two passions: art and sports. Hofmekler's formative experience as a young man with the Israeli Special Forces, prompted a lifetime's interest in diets and fitness regimes that would optimize his physical and mental performance.

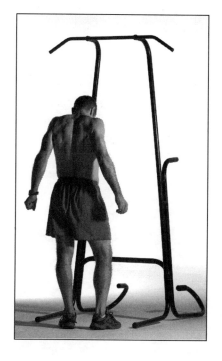

After the army, Ori attended the Bezalel Academy of Art and the Hebrew University, where he studied art and philosophy and received a degree in Human Sciences.

A world-renowned painter, best known for his controversial political satire, Ori's work has been featured in magazines worldwide, including *Time, Newsweek, Rolling Stone, People, The New Republic* as well as *Penthouse* where he was a monthly columnist for 17 years and Health Editor from 1998–2000. Ori has published two books of political art, *Hofmekler's People*, and *Hofmekler's Gallery*.

As founder, Editor-In-Chief, and Publisher of *Mind & Muscle POWER*, a national men's health and fitness magazine, Ori introduced his Warrior Diet to the public in a monthly column—to immediate acclaim from readers and professionals in the health industry alike.

REFERENCES

Airola, P. *Every Woman's book*, Health Plus Publishers, 1979.

Atkins, R. *Dr. Atkins – Age Defying Diet Revolution.* St. Martin's Press, 2000.

Atkins, R. *New Diet Revolution*, Avon Books, 1992.

Atkins, R. *Vita Nutrient Solution*, Simon & Schuster, 1998.

Atkins, R., Herwood, R. W. *Dr. Atkins's Diet Revolution.* Bantam, 1972.

Avery, S. *The Dimensional Structure of Consciousness, A Physical Basis for Immaterialism.* Compari.

Colbin, A.M. *Food and Healing.* Ballantine Books, 1986, 1996.

Cousens, G. *Conscious Eating.* North Atlantic Books, 2000.

Cousens, G. *Depression-Free For Life.* William Morrow, 2000.

Cousens, G. *Spiritual Nutrition and The Rainbow Diet*, North Atlantic Books, 1986.

D'Adamo, P., Whitney, C. *Eat Right For Your Type.* G.P. Putnam's Sons, 1996.

Diamond, H. *Fit For Life: A New Beginning*, Kensington Books, 2000.

Diamond, H., Diamond, M. *Fit For Life*, Warner, 1987.

Diamond, J. *Guns, Germs, and Steel-The Fates of Human Societies*, Norton, 1999

Dupont, F. *Daily Life In Ancient Rome.* Blackwell, 1993.

Erasmus, U. *Fats That Heal, Fats That Kill.* Alive Books, 1986, 1993.

Erdkamp, P. *Hunger and the Sword.* Gieben, 1998.

Garnsey, P. Cities, *Peasants, and Food in Classical Antiquity.* Cambridge University Press.

Giacosa, I. G. *A Taste Of Ancient Rome.* University of Chicago Press, 1992

Hamilton, E. *Mythology.* Massada Ltd. Israel, 1982

Hass, E.M., Stauth, C. *The False Fat Diet.* Ballantine Books, 2000.

Jensen, B. *Foods That Heal.* Avery, 1988, 1993.

Karch, B. *Herbal Medicine.* Advanced Research Press, 1999.

Murray, M.T. *Encyclopedia of Nutritional Supplements.* Prima Health, 1996.

Murray, M.T. *The Healing Power of Herbs.* Prima Health, 1992,1995.

Pliny the Elder (Naturalis Historia)

Plutarch. *Greeks.* Bialik Institute, Jerusalem, 1986

Sears, B. Lawren, B. *Enter The Zone*, Regan Books, 1995.

Solomon, J. 1950. *Ancient Roman Feasts and Recipes Adapted For Modern Cooking*. Seemann Pub, 1977.

Spark, R. *Sexual Health For Men*. Perseus Books, 2000.

Wagner, D. and Cousens, G. *Tachyon Energy* North Atlantic Books, 1999.

Weil, A. *Eating Well For Optimum Health*. Alfred A. Knopf, 2000.

Weil, A. *Natural Health Natural Medicine*. Houghton Mifflin Company, 1995.

Weil, A. *Spontaneous Healing*. Alfred A Knopf, Inc., 1995.

Additional Research Materials/Sources:

Andriamampandry MD, et al. Centre d'Ecologie et Physiologie Energetiques, Strasbourg, France. "Food deprivation modifies fatty acid partitioning and beta-oxidation capacity in rat liver." J Nutr 1996 Aug; 126(8): 2020-7.

Beck B, Stricker-Krongrad A, Burlet A, Nicolas JP, Burlet C. "Specific hypothalamic neuropeptide Y variation with diet parameters in rats with food choice." Neuroreport 1992 Jul; 3(7): 571-4

Benthem L, van der Leest J, Steffens AB, Zijlstra WG. Department of Medical Physiology, University of Groningen, The Netherlands. "Metabolic and hormonal responses to adrenoceptor antagonists in 48-hour-starved exercising rats." Metabolism 1995 Oct; 44(10): 1332-9.

Bereket A, Wilson TA, Kolasa AJ, Fan J, Lang CH. Department of Pediatrics, State University of New York, Stony Brook. "Regulation of the insulin-like growth factor system by acute acidosis." Endocrinology 1996 Jun; 137(6): 2238-45.

Bergstrom J, Hermansen L, Hultman E, Saltin B. "Diet, muscle glycogen and physical performance." Acta Physiol. Scand. 71: 140-150, 1967.

Bogardus C, LaGrange BM, Horton ES, Sims EA. "Comparison of carbohydrate-containing and carbohydrate-restricted hypocaloric diets in the treatment of obesity." "Endurance and metabolic fuel homeostasis during strenuous exercise." J Clin Invest 1981 Aug; 68(2):399-404.

Brun S, et al. Departament de Bioquimica I Biologia Molecular, Universitat de Barcelona, Spain. "Uncoupling protein-3 gene expression in skeletal muscle during development is regulated by nutritional factors that alter circulating non-esterified fatty acids." FEBS Lett 1999 Jun 18; 453(1-2): 205-9.

Cai XJ, et al. "Hypothalamic orexin expression: modulation by blood glucose and feeding." Diabetes 1999 Nov; 48(11): 2132-7.

Clark MG, et al. "Hypertension in obesity may reflect a homeostatic thermogenic response." Life Sci 1991; 48(10): 939-47.

Coleman, E. "Carbohydrates: the master fuel." In: Sports Nutrition for the 90's, eds. Berning, JR and Stenn, SN. Aspen Publishers, 1991.

Conlee RE. "Muscle glycogen and exercise endurance: a twenty year perspective." Exercise and Sports Science Reviews (1987) 15: 1-28.

Costill DL, Sherman WM, Fink WWJ Witten MW, Miller JM. "The role of dietary carbohydrates in muscle glycogen resynthesis after strenuous running." Am.J Clin. Nutr. 34: 1831-1836, 1981.

Covasa M, Ritter RC. "Rats maintained on high-fat diets exhibit reduced satiety in response to CCK and bombesin." Peptides 1998; 19(8): 1407-15.

Davis - Nutrition Department, University of California. "Effective nutritional ergogenic aids." Int J Sport Nutr 1999 Jun; 9(2):229-39.

Deferrari G, Garibotto G, Robaudo C, Saffioti S, Russo R, Sofia A. Department of Internal Medicine, University of Genoa, Italy. "Protein and amino acid metabolism in splanchnic organs in metabolic acidosis." Miner Electrolyte Metab 1997; 23(3-6):229-33.

Dulloo AG, Jacquet J, Girardier L. University of Geneva, Switzerland. "Autoregulation of body composition during weight recovery in human: the Minnesota Experiment revisited." Int J Obes Relat Metab Disord 1996 May; 20(5): 393-405.

Evans SJ, LoHC, Ney DM, Welbourne TC. Department of Nutritional Sciences, University of Wisconsin. "Acid-base homeostasis parallels anabolism in surgically stressed rats treated with GH and IGF-I." Am J Physiol 1996 Jun; 270(6 Pt 1): E968-74.

Forslund AH, et al. Department of Medical Sciences and Nutrition, Uppsala University, Uppsala, Sweden. "Effect of protein intake and physical activity on 24-h pattern and rate of macronutrient utilization." Am J Physiol 1999 May; 276(5Pt 1):E964-76.

Hagan MM, Havel PJ, Seely RJ, Woods SC, Ekhator NN, et al. Department of Psychiatry, University of Cincinnati College of Medicine. "Cerebrospinal fluid and plasma leptin measurements: covariability with dopamine and cortisol in fasting humans." J Clin Endocrinol Metab 1999 Oct; 84(10): 3579-85.

Heinz Rupp, Ph.D. "Hypercaloric nutrition, sympathetic activity and hypertension." Editorial to the Symposium "The Excess Catecholamine Syndrome. From Cause To Therapy."

Hocman, G. "Prevention of cancer: restriction of nutritional energy intake (joules)." Comp Biochem Physiol A 1988; 91(2):209-20

Holness MJ, Sugden MC. Department of Biochemistry, London Hospital Medical College, UK. "Pyruvate dehydrogenase activities and rates of lipogenesis during the fed-to-starved transition in liver and brown adipose tissue of the rat." Biochem J 1990 May 15; 268(1):77-81.

Isidori AM, et al. "Leptin and androgens in male obesity: evidence for leptin contribution to reduced androgen levels." J Clin Endocrinol Metab 1999 Oct; 84(10): 3673-80.

Jones BS, Yeaman, SJ, Sugden MC, Holness MJ. Department of Biochemistry and Genetics, Medical School, University of New Castle-upon-Tyne, UK. "Hepatic pyruvate dehydrogenase kinase activities during the starved-to-fed transition." Biochim Biophys Acta 1992 Mar 16; 1134(2): 164-8.

Kersten S, et al. Institute de Biologie Animale, Universite de Lausanne, Switzerland. Department de Physiologie, Faculte de Medecine, Universite de Geneve, Laboratory of Metabolism, National Cancer Institute. "Peroxisome proliferator-activated receptor alpha mediates the adaptive response to fasting." J Clin Invest 1999Jun; 103(11): 1489-98

Lambert EV et. al. "Enhanced endurance in trained cyclists during moderate intensity exercise following 2 weeks adaptation to a high fat diet." Eur J Apply Phyiol (1994) 69: 387-293.

Levin BE, Sullivan AC. "Regulation of thermogenesis in obesity." Int J Obes 1984; 8 Suppl 1:159-80.

Ludwig DS, et al. "High glycemic index foods, overeating, and obesity." Pediatrics 1999 Mar; 103(3): E26.

Marti A., Berraondo B, Martinez JA. "Leptin: physiological actions." J Physiol Biochem 1999 Mar; 55(1)43-9.

Metabolism 1983 Aug; 32(8):769-76.

Minassian C, Montana S, Mithieux G. "Regulatory role of glucose-6 phosphatase in the repletion of liver glycogen during refeeding in fasted rats." Biochim Biophys Acta 1999 Nov 11;1452(2): 172-8.

Newby FD, Wilson LK, Thacker SV, DiGirolamo M. Department of Medicine, Emory University School of Medicine. "Adipocyte lactate production remains elevated during refeeding after fasting." Am J Physiol 1990 Dec; 259(6 Pt 1): E865-71.

O'Dea K, et al. "Noradrenaline turnover during under- and over-eating in normal weight subjects." Metabolism 1982 Sep; 31(9):896-9.

Ogihara H, et al. Gunma U"niversity School of Medicine, Maebashi, Japan. "Peptide transporter in the rat small intestine: ultrastructural localization and the effect of starvation and administration of amino acids." Histochem J 1999 Mar; 31(3): 169-74.

Phinney S. "Exercise during and after very-low-calorie dieting." Am J Clin Nutr (1992) 56: 190S-194S.

Phinney SD et. al. "Effects of aerobic exercise on energy expenditure and nitrogen balance during very low calorie dieting." Metabolism (1988) 37: 758-765.

Phinney SD, Bistrian BR, Evans WJ, Gervino E, Blackburn GL. "The human metabolic response to chronic ketosis without caloric restriction: preservation of submaximal exercise capability with reduced oxidation." Metabolism (1983) 32: 769-776.

Plata-Salaman CR. "Regulation of hunger and satiety in man." Dig Dis 1991; 9(5): 253-68.

Radomski MW, Cross M, Buguet A. Defense and Civil Institute of Environmental Medicine, North York, ON, Canada. "Exercise-induced hyperthermia and hormonal responses to exercise." Can J Physiol Pharmacol 1998 May; 76(5): 547-52.

Reuters. "Mice That Overexpress Human UCP-3 Eat More Yet Weigh Less Than Wild-Type Mice." July 27, 2000.

Samec S, Seydoux J, Dulloo AG. "Inter-organ signaling between adipose tissue metabolism and skeletal muscle uncoupling protein homologs: is there a role for circulating free fatty acids?" Diabetes 1998 Nov; 47(11): 1693-8.

Sandberg PR. "Carbohydrate loading and deploying forces." Bravo Company, 2nd Battalion, 3rd Special Forces Group (Airborne), Fort Bragg, NC 28307, USA. Mil Med 1999 Sep; 164(9): 636-42.

Schreihofer DA, Parfitt DB, Cameron JL. "Suppression of luteinizing hormone secretion during short-term fasting in male rhesus monkeys: the role of metabolic versus stress signals." Department of Behavioral Neuroscience, University of Pittsburgh, Pennsylvania. Endocrinology 1993 May; 132(5): 1881-9

Selvais PL, et al. "Cyclic feeding behavior and changes in hypothalamic galanin and neuropeptide Y gene expression induced by zinc deficiency in the rat. J Neuroendocrinol 1997 Jan; 9(1): 55-62.

Sherman WM, Coastal DJ, Fink WJ Miller JM. "Effect of exercise-diet manipulation on muscle glycogen supercompensation and its subsequent utilization during performance." Int. J. Sports Med. 2:114-118, 1981.

Sherman, W. "Carbohydrates, muscle glycogen, and muscle glycogen supercompensation." In: Ergogenic Aids in Sports, ed. Williams, M. Human Kinetics Publishers, 1983.

Sivitz WI, Fink BD, Donohue PA. Department of Internal Medicine, University of Iowa and the Iowa City Veterans Affairs Medical Center. "Fasting and leptin modulate adipose and muscle uncoupling protein: divergent effects between messenger ribonucleic acid and protein expression." Endocrinology 1999 Apr; 140(4): 1511-9.

Strack AM, Akana SF, Horsley CJ, Dallman MF. Department of Physiology, University of California, San Francisco. "A hypercaloric load induces thermogenesis but inhibits stress responses in the SNS and HPA system." Am J Physiol 1997 Mar; 272(3 Pt 2):R840-8.

Svanberg, Elizabeth, et al. University Hospital, University of Goteborg, Sweden, College of Medicine, Pennsylvania State University. "Postprandial stimulation of muscle protein synthesis is mediated through translation initiation and is independent of changes in insulin." APStracts 19 February 1997.

Wang J, Leibowitz KL. "Central insulin inhibits hypothalamic galanin and neuropeptide Y gene expression and peptide release in intact rats." Brain Res 1997 Nov 28; 777(1-2):231-6.

Welbourne TC, Milford L, Carter P. Department of Molecular and Cellular Physiology, Lousiana State University Medical Center. "The role of growth hormone in substrate utilization." Baillieres Clin Endocrinol Metab 1997 Dec; 11 (4):699-707.

ADDITIONAL
RESOURCES

Harvey Diamond is the bestselling author of *Fit For Life*, which has sold 12 million copies worldwide, and has been translated into thirty-two languages. He has been writing and lecturing on health and nutrition for the last thirty years. His latest book, *Fit For Life: A New Beginning*, was published in June 2000. If you would like to learn more about Harvey Diamond and *Fit For Life*, call toll free: 877-335-1509 or visit www.hdiamond.com.

INDEX

A

abdominal exercises, 208–218
  crunches, 214–217
  final leg raise, 217
  hanging leg raise, 213–214
  lower-back stretch, 218
  principles behind, 207–209, 211–213
  "Warrior Posture" and, 209–211
acid-base balance, 92, 157–158
acupuncture, 11
adaptation period, 16, 26–27
ADD. See Attention Deficit Disorder (ADD)
adenosylemethionine (SAMe), 111, 112
adipose tissue, 103. See also body fat
aerobic training, 259–265
  bicycling/stationary biking, 264–265
  goals of, 260
  principles behind, 192, 203, 259, 261
  sprint intervals, 261–264
aggressive instinct, 168
alcohol
  beer, 134

body fat and, 106, 108, 110, 113, 185
cravings for, 185
determining intake of, 106, 108, 185
estrogenic effects of, 91, 106
in Greco-Roman culture, 135, 138
illnesses caused by, 106, 178, 185
sexual functioning and, 304
vitamin deficiencies and, 41
wine, 91, 134, 135, 185, 304
Alexander the Great, 127, 130, 135, 139, 147
alfalfa sprouts, 67
algae, 173
allergies
body fat and, 106, 107, 113
case study about, 310–312
to corn, 95
to dairy, 72, 90, 95
detoxification and, 24–25
diagnosis of, 95
eating frequency and, 11
to eggs, 74, 95
enzyme supplements and, 38
to nuts, 79, 80, 95
to protein, 74

bananas, 139

barbecuing/grilling, 74, 280–282

barbell front raise, 240

barley, 84, 142

beans, 73, 141–144

bee pollen, 173

beer, 134

beets, 83, 172–173

benign prostate hyperplasia (BPH), 178, 179

berries, 31–32, 41, 56, 66, 84, 289, 292

beverages

    alcohol. See alcohol

    coffee, 20, 31, 61, 205

    consumption during Overeating Phase, 58, 59–60

    consumption during Undereating Phase, 20, 31

    juices, 29–30, 31, 93, 172

    milk, 31, 45

    need for, 59–60

    packaging of, 106, 107, 108

    soft drinks, 31

    tea, 20, 31, 60, 61, 205

    water. See water

biceps exercises, 256, 258

bicycling/stationary biking, 264–265

bingeing, 5, 150, 158–159, 309

blue-green algae, 173

body fat, 103–113

    alcohol intake and, 106, 108, 110, 113, 185

    allergies and, 106, 107, 113

    burning of, 16, 17, 25, 26, 36–37, 38, 83, 103–104, 108–112, 121, 122, 159–160, 164, 206

    carbohydrate consumption and, 83, 103–105, 106, 108

    development of, 11, 103–108

    dieting and. See diets/ dieting; weight loss

    eating frequency and, 11, 163

    enzyme supplements and, 36–37, 38

    estrogen and, 104, 105, 106, 107, 108–109, 112, 113

    exercise and, 106–107, 108, 113, 125

    insulin insensitivity and, 104–105

    lipase deficiency and, 36–37, 38

    in men, 105, 161–162

    metabolism and, 103–104

    muscle building and, 162

    nutrition and, 105, 108–112

    Overeating Phase and, 51, 59, 159–160

    preventing development of, 106–108

    protein consumption and, 105

    recommended amount of, 161–162

    stress and, 105

supplements and, 108–112

surgical removal of, 103

water intake and, 113

in women, 105, 310

bodybuilders. See also athletes

dietary needs of, 117

muscle building and, 162

protein consumption by, 34

training of. See training program

water retention by, 94

bow-and-arrow stretch, 241–242

BPH. See benign prostate hyperplasia (BPH)

Bragg, Paul, 22

"brain boosters," 43–44

"brain-power factor," 157

breast cancer, 170

broccoli, 66

Buchinger, Dr., 22

buckwheat, 84

butter, 77

C

Caesar. See Julius Caesar

caffeine, 20, 31, 42, 205

calcium supplements, 37, 39–40

calf stretching, 221

calories, 159, 160

cancer

alcohol intake and, 106

barbecuing/grilling meat and, 4

in children, 169

eating habits and, 22, 24, 73

environmental toxins and, 169–170

enzyme supplements and, 38

fermented foods and, 90

fiber consumption and, 73, 89

nitric oxide and, 188

nut consumption and, 78, 79

radiation and, 170–171

types of. See specific cancers

canola oil, 76

Carbohydrate Addict's Diet, 150

carbohydrates, 81–88

athletes' consumption of, 153, 161

body fat and, 83, 103–105, 106, 108

complex vs. simple, 81–82, 153

consumption during Overeating Phase, 55, 81–88, 153

consumption during Undereating Phase, 17, 20, 35–36, 85

cooking of, 82

daily intake of, 82

depletion of, 152

diets high in, 118, 120–121

diets low in, 118, 122–124, 150, 152

effects of consuming, 82–83, 93

D

D'Adamo, Peter, 79, 86

daily food cycle. See Warrior
Cycle

dairy, 71–72
 allergies to, 72, 90, 95
 cheese, 71–72
 contamination of, 178
 fat content of, 33, 45, 71–72,
 77, 87
 fermented types of, 90
 in Greco-Roman diet, 143
 organic, 71
 types of, 71–72

dairy protein powders, 46

dandelion root, 111, 112

dead lifts, 248–249

dehydration, 59–60

dehydro-testosterone (DHT),
175–176, 178, 179

dematerialization, 11

depression, 22, 121

desserts
 with main meal, 87–88
 recipes for, 286–292

detoxification, 22–26, 117
 allergies and, 24–25
 effects of, 22–25
 healing process and, 24–25
 immune system and, 24
 nature of, 23, 308
 routine for, 172

Undereating Phase and, 12,
16, 17, 22–26, 48
 for women, 308

DHT. See dehydro-testosterone

Diamond, Harvey, 118, 124,
125–126

diets/dieting, 115–126. See also
body fat; weight loss
 age and, 182, 183–184
 body fat and, 106, 113
 business events and, 184
 carbohydrates and, 118,
 122–124, 150, 152
 cycle of weight loss/gain,
 106, 107, 113, 307–308
 detoxification and, 123, 124,
 126
 freedom and, 163–164
 healing as element in, 118,
 124–125
 live/living foods and, 122,
 123, 124, 125, 126, 168–169
 overeating syndrome,
 158–159
 protein in, 118, 120–121,
 122–124
 salt intake and, 94–95
 sexual functioning and,
 300–301, 305
 social events and, 184
 stability of, 115–116
 supplement use and, 122,
 123
 types of, 116, 117, 118–126.

See also specific types

women and, 307–308

digestion

acid-base balance and, 92, 157–158

of cooked foods, 64–65, 67

enzymes involved in, 30, 32, 38

of fermented foods, 89

fiber consumption and, 89, 93, 139, 173

food separation and, 126

of live/living foods, 56, 64

problems with, 24, 67–68, 89 92, 117, 139, 158

wine as aid to, 91

disease. See healing process; illness/illnesses

DMAE, 43–44

dopamine, 44, 73, 205, 305

drugs

alcohol. See alcohol

for animals, 7

marijuana, 178

overuse of, 25

sexual functioning and, 299

E

eating habits

bingeing, 5, 150, 158–159, 309

cancer and, 22, 24, 73

of classical hunters, 2

diets/dieting. See

diets/dieting

energy and, 11, 13, 158

fasting. See fasting

frequency, 11, 63, 117, 158, 160, 163

of Hunters vs. Scavengers, 6–7

instinct for, 52, 54, 58, 158–160, 183

metabolism and, 156

overeating, 158–159. See also Overeating Phase

sleep and, 13

undereating. See Undereating Phase

toxins and, 11, 12, 22

echinacea, 174

EFAs. See essential fatty acids (EFAs)

egg-protein powders, 48

eggplant, 68

eggs, 70–71

allergies to, 74, 95

cholesterol content of, 71

cooking of, 274

eating with other foods, 67–68

organic, 48

as protein source, 70–71

recipes for, 274–279

sulfur content of, 67–68

elimination (of body wastes), 23, 24. See also digestion

"empty stomach factor," 43, 44.
See also exercise, on empty
stomach
energy
eating habits and, 11, 13, 158
excessive levels of, 186
mental, 43–44, 150, 157
physical, 9
spiritual nature of, 9, 10
in Undereating Phase, 11, 13,
17–18, 22, 25, 26, 48, 157
environmental toxins, 169–174.
See also toxins
enzyme loading, 36
enzymes
allergies and, 38
antiaging and, 36
body fat and, 36–37, 38
cancer and, 38
digestion and, 30, 32, 38
effects of, 36
in live/living foods, 30
nature of, 22, 24
need for, 186
protein utilization and, 35
supplements, 186, 187–189,
319
types of, 38
Erasmus, Udo, 107, 109
essential fatty acids (EFAs), 48,
70, 74, 75–76, 120–121, 270
Ester C, 41
estrogen, 45, 47
body fat and, 104, 105, 106,

107, 108–109, 112, 113
derivatives of, 169, 170
prostate cancer and, 175–176
estrogenic foods/substances,
177–178
alcohol, 106
avoiding consumption of,
106
blocking effects of, 66,
108–110, 112
body fat and, 104, 106, 113
chemical and environmental
toxins, 169–171, 175–176
plastic, 107
prostate problems and, 177
soy, 47, 108–109
wheat, 86
whey protein, 45
wine, 91
exercise. See also training
program
body fat and, 106–107, 108,
113, 125
caffeine consumption before,
205
daily food intake and, 181
on empty stomach, 161, 164,
181, 203, 205, 206, 266
foods to consume
before/after, 99, 164,
203–207, 266
frequency of, 181
in Greco-Roman culture,
191–192
hunger and, 181

mineral supplements and, 39
  sexual functioning and, 302
  stress and, 113
  supplement use and, 39, 41
  after Undereating Phase, 48
  for women, 267–268

F

falconry, 3–5
false romanticism, 166–168.
  See also Romantic Instinct
fast food, 56, 118, 119, 183
fasting
  breaking from, 19
  controlled, 4, 17–22. See also
  Undereating Phase
  effects of, 17–18
  instinct and, 22
  spiritual aspects of, 20, 21,
  157, 186
  starvation vs., 20–21
  types of, 17
fat
  in avocados, 36–37
  in butter, 77
  in dairy, 33, 45, 71–72, 77,
  87
  denaturation of, 30
  diets low in, 118, 120–121,
  163
  essential fatty acids (EFAs),
  48, 70, 74, 75–76, 120–121,
  270
  on meat, 68, 69
  need for, 74, 76

in nuts, 36–37, 77, 78, 79
in oils, 74–77, 142, 143
in overprocessed foods, 55
in seeds, 80
sugar and, 87–88
transfatty acids, 77
fermented foods, 89–92. See
also specific foods
fertilizers, 169–170, 178
fiber
  benefits of consuming, 89,
  93, 173
  cancer prevention and, 73, 89
  in carbohydrates, 83, 93
  in cooked vegetables, 66, 67
  digestion and, 89, 93, 139,
  173
  insulin levels and, 89
  in legumes, beans, and peas,
  73
final leg raise, 217
fish, 69–70
  contamination of, 69–70
  in Greco-Roman diet, 143
  oils contained in, 69–70
  as protein source, 69–70
  recipes for, 272, 282
Fit for Life diet, 118, 124,
125–126
flat bench barbell press, 245,
246–247
flavones, 64, 66, 123
flaxseed oil, 75
food separation, 126

glycogen, 53, 161

goldenseal, 174

grains, 84–87

  benefits of consuming, 66–67

  as carbohydrate source, 84–87

  diets high in, 124, 141, 142

  in Greco-Roman diet, 141, 142

  types of, 84–86, 142. See also specific types

grape seed extract, 41

grape seed extract, 41

grapes, 94

Greco-Roman culture, 127–149

  alcohol in, 135, 138

  applications to modern culture/diet, 147–149

  class divisions in, 131, 132, 134, 135, 139, 141–142, 143–144, 146

  daily activities in, 132–133

  exercise in, 191–192

  food in, 133–138, 141–144

  as foundation of Western civilization, 127

  health issues in, 139–141

  self-image in, 127, 128–129, 191–192

  soldiers in, 127–133, 143–145

  values of, 127, 128–131

  world domination by, 128, 144–145

  yearly cycle of, 131–132

Greeks. See Greco-Roman culture

grilling, 74, 280–282

growth factors, 44, 45

growth hormone (GH), 17–18

guarana, 205

H

hack squats, 227

hamstring stretch, 256

hanging leg raise, 213–214

health/healing

  controlled fasting and, 22, 24–25

  detoxification and, 24–25

  diets/dieting and, 118, 124–125, 168–169

  exercise. See exercise; training program

  in Greco-Roman culture, 139–141

  homeopathic remedies, 78, 140, 172–175, 180, 280

  nature of, 11–12

  sexual functioning. See sexual functioning

  supplements and, 42, 178–180. See also supplements

herbicides, 169–170, 178

Scavenger, 1, 5, 6

sexual, 293–296, 303–304.
See also sexual functioning

Survivor/Multiplier, 1, 2

Warrior, 1–7

Instinctive Healing diet, 118, 124, 125

insulin

body fat and, 104–105, 106, 108

carbohydrate consumption and, 82, 83, 93–94, 104–105, 106, 108, 120, 162–163

controlled fasting and, 17, 21, 25, 26

fiber consumption and, 89

glucagon vs., 121

monitoring levels of, 31, 82, 83, 93–94

sugar consumption and, 31

insulin insensitivity, 104–105, 120, 153, 161, 162–163

intense resistance training, 195–197

iodized salt. See also sodium

ionized mineral supplements, 18

IP6 (inositol hexaphosphate), 66–67, 73

iron oxidation, 45

J

juices, 29–30, 31, 93, 172

Julius Caesar, 127, 132, 135, 147, 149

junk food, 56, 118, 119

K

kamut, 86

L

lactic-acid efficiency, 200–201

lactoferin, 45

lateral pull-downs, 242–243

laterals, 234, 238–239

lecithin, 81, 270

leg (knee) extensions, 220

leg curls, 223

leg exercises, 219–229

back squats, 225–227

calf stretching, 221

front squats, 224–225

hack squats, 227

leg (knee) extensions, 220

leg curls, 223

lunges, 227–228

principles behind, 219–220

sissy squats, 229

standing calf raises, 221, 222

superset, 223

legumes, 66–67, 73

lentils, 66–67, 73

leukemia, 169

lignans, 109–110, 112

lipase deficiency, 36–37, 38, 77

liposuction, 103

live/living foods, 29–30
consumption during Overeating Phase, 56–57
consumption during Undereating Phase, 16, 18, 64
diets high in, 125, 126, 168–169
diets low in, 122, 123, 124
digestion of, 56, 64
effects of eating, 18, 30
enzymes in, 30
minerals in, 32–33
types of, 16, 18, 29–30
liver detoxifiers, 110–112
lower-back stretch, 218
lunges, 227–228
lysine, 105

M

macrobiotic diets, 118, 124–125
magnesium deficiency, 40
main meal, 63–101. See also Overeating Phase
carbohydrates in, 81–89. See also carbohydrates
cooking foods for, 63–67, 73–74, 82
fruits in, 83–84. See also fruits
protein in, 69–74. See also protein
selecting foods for, 63, 65–66, 67, 69, 98, 101
time eaten, 59, 61
vegetables in, 65–69. See also vegetables

margarine, 77
marijuana, 178
meat. See also fish; poultry
barbecuing/grilling of, 74, 280–282
contamination of, 169–170, 177
cooking of, 73–74, 270
fat content of, 68, 69
fruit combined with, 81–82
in Greco-Roman diet, 142
organic, 7, 69
as protein source, 69–70
recipes for, 271–273, 280–282
sexual functioning and eating of, 70
melatonin, 151
men
body fat in, 105, 161–162
sexual performance of, 70, 296. See also sexual functioning
mental acuity, 43–44, 150, 157
metabolism
body fat and, 103–104
of carbohydrates, 17, 93
eating and rate of, 156
efficiency of, 53, 54, 151, 156, 159–160
Overeating Phase and, 159–160
milk, 31, 45, 87, 205

overacidity, 92, 117

Overeating Phase, 51–61, 63–101

   beverage consumption during, 58, 59–60

   body fat and, 51, 59, 159–160

   calorie consumption during, 160

   carbohydrate consumption during, 55, 81–88, 153

   by classical hunters, 2–3

   cycling diet and, 4, 155–157

   effects of, 11, 53, 54

   exercising before, 181

   foods for, 52, 55–60, 63–101, 98. See also main meal

   fruit consumption during, 56–57

   goals of, 53

   metabolism and, 159–160

   principles behind, 51–52, 53, 54, 308–309

   protein consumption during, 55

   reaching satiety, 58, 59–60, 158–159

   vegetable consumption during, 55, 56

   water consumption during, 60

   women and, 308–309

overeating syndrome, 158–159

P

packaging materials, 106, 107, 108, 113

panax, 42. See also ginseng

partial-press reps, 252

pasta, 93

pasteurization, 46, 72

pastries, 95–96

peanuts, 79, 95

pears, 32

peas, 73

pesticides, 169–170, 178

physical attraction, 293–296

pickled foods, 90

pine nuts, 79

pistachios, 80

pizza, 65

plants and roots, 83

plastic

   derivatives of, 169, 170

   as packaging material, 106, 107, 108, 113

Pliny the Elder, 143

Plutarch, 129

polyunsaturated oils, 76

potassium, 94–95

potatoes, 83, 93

Pottenger Cat Study, 297–299

poultry, 143, 271, 281

predators, 3–5. See also Hunter/Predator Instinct

preworkout meals, 203–205

probiotics, 30, 34–35, 39, 89

prolactin, 44, 45, 175, 176
prostate cancer, 170
prostate enlargement, 175–180
protein, 69–74
  allergies to, 74
  athletes'/bodybuilders' consumption of, 34, 44
  body fat and, 105
  consumption during Overeating Phase, 55
  consumption during Undereating Phase, 20, 33–35
  cooking of, 73–74
  cravings for, 69
  denaturation of, 34, 46, 74
  diets high in, 118, 122–124
  diets low in, 118, 120–121
  enzyme loading and, 35
  foods containing, 69–74. See also specific foods
  in Greco-Roman diet, 142–143
  in main meal, 69–74
  organic sources of, 70
  sulfur content of, 67–68
  in vegetables, 173
protein powders, 33, 44–48
Protein Power Diet, 150
protein utilization, 34–35, 72–73, 318
pull-ups, 234–237, 240
pumpkin seeds, 80
pumpkins, 83, 287
pygeum, 178–179

Q

quercetin, 109, 112
quinoa, 85

R

radiation, 170–173
Ramadan, 186
recovery meals, 203, 206–207
resistance training, 194–203
  back strength, 194
  controlled fatigue, 198–200
  cycling of activities, 195–196
  high-velocity, 195–196, 197–198
  intense resistance, 195–197
  joint strength, 194–195
  lactic-acid efficiency, 200–201
  length of workout, 202–203
  principles of, 193
  reaching failure, 201–202
rice, 84, 93
Romans. See Greco-Roman culture
Romantic Instinct, 164–168

S

safflower oil, 76
salt. See sodium
SAMe. See adenosylemethionine (SAMe)
saturated oils, 76–77
saw palmetto, 178, 179

spirituality, 9, 10, 20, 21, 157, 186

sports. See athletes; exercise; training program

sprint intervals, 261–264

sprouted wheat, 86

squash, 68, 83

standing barbell press, 232–233

standing calf raises, 221, 222

starches, 87–88. See also carbohydrates

starvation, 20–21

steroids, 111, 170

stinging nettle, 110, 112

strength training. See resistance training

stress

body fat and, 105

carbohydrate consumption and, 151

eating frequency and, 158

exercise and, 113

ginseng and, 42

glutamine and, 43

mineral supplements and, 39–40

sexual functioning and, 296, 301

vitamin supplements and, 41

stubborn fat, 103–113. See also body fat

causes of, 104–105

elimination of, 108–112, 113

nature of, 103–104

prevention of, 106–108, 113

sugar

allergies to, 95

consumption during Undereating Phase, 20

content in fruit, 31–32, 84

cravings for, 88, 150, 183

fat and, 87–88

negative effects of consuming, 24, 55, 95–96, 122, 153

sulfur, 67–68, 173

sunflower oil, 76

sunflower seeds, 80

super oxide dismutase (SOD), 188

supplements. See also Warrior Diet Nutritional Supplements

athletes' consumption of, 38

criticism of use of, 168–169

diets including use of, 122, 123

enzyme, 186, 187–189, 319

exercise and, 39, 41

fat burning, 108–112

mineral, 39–40, 171–172

prostate enlargement treatments, 178–180

for Undereating Phase, 37–43, 49

vitamin, 41

Survivor/Multiplier Instinct, 1, 2

sweets, 87–88. See also carbohydrates; desserts; sugar

sympathetic nervous system (SNS), 157–158

T

tea, 20, 31, 60, 61, 205
teenagers, 183–184
tendon stretch, 232
thirst, 58, 59–60, 96
thyroid, 151, 301
tomatoes, 66
toxins, 169–174
    eating habits and, 11, 12, 22
    elimination of. See detoxification
    estrogenic derivatives, 169, 170
    illnesses caused by, 22–23, 169–170
    pesticides, herbicides, and fertilizers, 169–170
    plastic derivatives, 169, 170
    protection from, 171–175
    radiation, 170–173
    raw plants and, 67
training program, 191–268
    abdominal exercises, 208–218
    aerobic element of, 192, 203, 259–265
    arm exercises, 256–258
    back and chest exercises, 242–249
    breathing properly, 208
    goals of, 191–192, 193
    hamstring stretch, 256
    high-velocity exercises, 197–198, 250–256
    leg exercises, 219–229
    preworkout meals, 203–205
    principles of, 193–202
    recovery meals, 203, 206–207
    resistance training element of, 193, 194–203
    shoulder exercises, 230–242
    water consumption and, 204
    for women, 267–268
transfatty acids, 77
tricep exercises, 256–257
tropical fruits, 32, 56–57, 84
Tyrosine, 43–44

U

Undereating Phase, 15–27, 29–48
    adaptation period of, 16, 26–27
    beverage consumption during, 20, 31
    carbohydrate consumption during, 17, 20, 35–36, 85
    by classical hunters, 2–3
    controlled fasting during, 4, 17–22
    cycling diet and, 4, 9, 10, 11, 155–157
    dematerialization and, 11
    detoxification and, 12, 16, 17, 22–26, 48
    effects of, 11, 12

Warrior Male Performance Support, 320–321

Warrior Milk, 72–73, 99, 101, 207, 316

"Warrior Posture," 209–211

Warrior Premier Norwegian Cod Liver Oil, 325

Warrior Probiotics, 317–318

Warrior Stubborn Fat Burner, 112, 322

Warrior-zyme, 188, 318–320

water
 body fat and, 113
 consumption during Overeating Phase, 60
 consumption during Undereating Phase, 20
 daily intake of, 31, 60, 97
 exercise and, 204
 glycogen and, 161
 metabolism and, 60
 purification of, 106, 107, 113

water fasts, 17, 27

water weight, 94

weight loss. See body fat; diets/dieting

Weil, Andrew, 118, 124, 125

wheat, 84, 86, 95, 142, 178

whey protein, 44–46, 72

whole foods, 168–169. See also live/living foods

whole grains, 81–82. See also carbohydrates

wine, 91, 134, 135, 185, 304

women, 307–312
 body fat in, 105, 310
 detoxification for, 308
 diets/dieting by, 307–308
 exercise for, 267–268
 hormonal fluctuations of, 111, 309
 Overeating Phase for, 308–309
 training program for, 267–268

working out. See exercise; training program

Y

yeast infections, 90

yin and yang, 124–125

yogurt, 292

yohimbe bark, 111–112

Yom Kippur, 186

Z

zinc, 40, 304

Zone, The (diet), 115, 118, 121–122, 150

ADDITIONAL RESOURCES

Harvey Diamond is the bestselling author of *Fit For Life*, which has sold 12 million copies worldwide, and has been translated into thirty-two languages. He has been writing and lecturing on health and nutrition for the last thirty years. His latest book, *Fit For Life: A New Beginning*, was published in June 2000. If you would like to learn more about Harvey Diamond and *Fit For Life*, call toll free: 877-335-1509 or visit www.hdiamond.com.

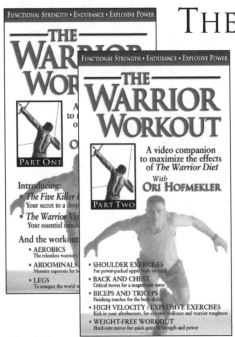

Praise for *The Warrior Workout* Videos

"Being a world class fighter, I can appreciate Ori's dedication and painstaking research in designing such a useful method of training. Ori and I share the same beliefs in functional strength training. Whether you are a novice or an elite athlete, the *Warrior Workout* videos are designed to guide you step by step to achieve your next level of physical and mental conditioning. It is inspiring to find someone who understands the true nature of a warrior's workout."
—**John R. Salgado, World Champion Shuai-Chiao (Chinese Wrestling), World Champion Taiji Push-Hands**

"The Warrior Workout videos are now a part of my fitness library. I believe Ori Hofmekler is right on target in his teaching of "functional strength". Using our basic instincts to train is what fitness should be about. If you are serious about being in your best physical shape, forget about "froo-froo" aerobics classes and less than optimal resistance training regimens. Train like a warrior. Tune your body in to its primal motivation for strength, then follow Ori's lead toward a stronger, healthier, and more vibrant you."
—**Laura Moore, Science writer, Penthouse Magazine, IronMan Magazine, Radio Talk Show Host "The Health Nuts", Body of the Month for IronMan Mag. Sept 2001**

"*The Warrior Workout* videos are a superb illustration of the power of the Warrior workout routine. They demonstrate the movements and skills necessary to rapidly carve the fat off your body and reveal lasting stone carved muscles."
—**Carlon M. Colker, M.D., F.A.C.N., author *The Greenwich Diet*, CEO and Medical Director, Peak Wellness, Inc., President and Founder, Peak Wellness Foundation**

"Ori Hofmekler has his finger on a deep, ancient and very visceral pulse—one that too many of us have all but forgotten. Part warrior-athlete, part philosopher-romantic, Ori not only reminds us what this innate, instinctive rhythm is all about, he also shows us how to detect and rekindle it in our own bodies. His *Warrior Workout* video program challenges and guides each of us to fully reclaim for ourselves the strength, sinew, energy and spirit that humans have always been meant to possess."
—**Pilar Gerasimo, Editor in Chief, Experience Life Magazine**

Discover:

- How to take advantage of controlled fatigue—and bust through to a new dimension of physical fitness
- How to "peak" your hormones—for maximum strength and fat loss
- How to pack greater gains into less time
- How the little-known secret of antagonistic-muscle synergy can turn a mediocre workout into a high-octane power-fest
- How to build a strong, lean body without using weights.

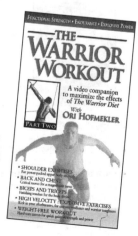

1•800•899•5111
24 HOURS A DAY FAX: (866)-280-7619

When Your Life is at Stake, You Owe it to Yourself to Get the Best

Warrior Growth Serum

Vanilla. 4.5 oz
#NWD01-VAN $49.95
Chocolate. 6 oz
#NWD01-CHOC $49.95

Adding *Growth Serum* to your diet is like jumping from a Yugo into a Ferrari. Yow! Prepare for neck-jerking G-Force and your hair flying in the wind.

Hardcore performance-athletes have hoarded the secret of colustrum's power-packed punch for as long as they can, but now we are breaking open the gates and letting you have at it.

But be warned, this is rocket-fuel for the body in its most exalted form and should not be used by the lame-at-heart or weak-kneed also-rans.

And be further warned: most colustrums being touted on the market today are treasonous for their pesticide-saturated, denatured, deadified slock that frankly ain't gonna do a darn thing for you but gunk you up and take your wallet to the cleaners.

So use what works! Feel the real thing fire you up and never look back.

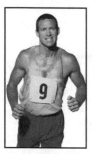

Warrior Growth Serum is a blend of undenatured air-dried colostrum produced from organically fed, drug-free, healthy cows, with other nutrients, such as grade A inulin and CLA, which support the metabolic system. This powder is high in immunosupportive protein, growth factors, and lactoferin—ingredients often missing in other dairy protein powders. *Warrior Growth Serum* is one magnificent potentiator—if you want that edge, how can you possibly be without it?

Warrior Male Performance Support

60 caps 600 mg #NWD04 $39.95

A blend of nutrients and herbs that naturally mimics the way testosterone works in the body. Warrior Male Performance Support contains:

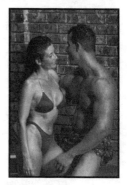

Testosterone Precursors—to enhance and accelerate testosterone production and synthesis. Vasodilators—to help ensure ample flow of blood and oxygen to every important part of the body. Cerebral supporters—to maintain healthy nerve impulses and hormonal balance in the brain.

In addition, Warrior Male Performance Support contains antioxidants, herbs, vitamins, proteins, and minerals to keep the mind and body naturally energized, support prostate health, and optimize sexual potency.

Warrior Milk

Vanilla 16 oz #NWD02-VAN $39.95
Chocolate 18 oz #NWD02-CHOC $39.95

A blend of specially processed, pesticide-free whey isolate, with growth serum and other nutrients that enhance its potency and assimilation. This protein powder can be used as a substitute for a cooked protein meal at times these foods aren't available. Warrior Milk should help you satisfy your daily protein requirement. Due to its protein composition, Warrior Milk is a great supplemental food for those interested in accelerating the anabolic process of building muscles.

Warrior Live Minerals

(capsules) 60 caps 880 mg
#NWD08A $29.95

The Warrior Minerals are derived from a once-living coral source. Coral minerals are highly ionized and contain the optimum ratio of calcium, magnesium, zinc, copper, and manganese, and other trace minerals. The ionic form of the Warrior Minerals is the most biologically active form, and the most absorbable. Ionized minerals help optimize the acid-base balance in your body. A healthy pH warrants healthy metabolism and overall health.

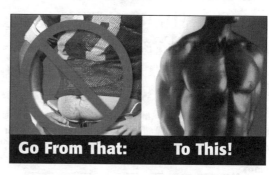

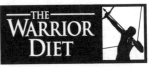

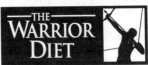

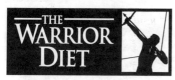

Supplement Order Form

Send your check or money order made out to:

Dragon Door Publications
PO Box 4381,
St. Paul, MN 55104

Item#	Qty.	Item Description	Price Ea.	Total
#NWD01-V		Warrior Growth Serum Vanilla—4.5 oz	$49.95	
#NWD01-C		Warrior Growth Serum Chocolate—6 oz.	$49.95	
#NWD02-V		Warrior Milk Vanilla—16 oz.	$39.95	
#NWD02-C		Warrior Milk Chocolate—18 oz.	$39.95	
#NWD03		Warrior Stubborn Fat Burner—45 caps 500 mg	$35.95	
#NWD04		Warrior Male Performance Support—60 caps 500 mg	$39.95	
#NWD08A		Warrior Live Minerals—60 caps 880 mg	$29.95	

Shipping address (if different from address on other side of this coupon)

Name:_____

Address:_____

City:_____ State: _____

Zip:_____ Phone:_____

e-mail:_____

HANDLING AND SHIPPING CHARGES

Total amount of order add:

$00.00	to	$24.99	add	$5.00
$25.00	to	$39.99	add	$6.00
$40.00	to	$59.99	add	$7.00
$60.00	to	$99.99	add	$10.00
$100.00	to	$129.99	add	$12.00
$130.00	to	$169.99	add	$14.00
$170.00	to	$199.99	add	$16.00
$200.00	to	$299.99	add	$18.00
$300.00	and up		add	$20.00

NO COD's

Total of Goods	
Discount Amount ($10 per item)	
Shipping Charges	
MN residents add 6.5% sales tax	
Total Enclosed	

Method of payment: ___Check ___M.O.

___Mastercard ___Visa ___Discover ___Amex

Account No. _____

Expiration Date_____Date_____

Signature _____

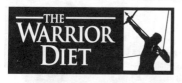

Supplement Order Form

If ordering by credit card call **1-800-899-5111**
If ordering by fax call **(866)-280-7619**
If ordering by e-mail, go to **dragondoor@aol.com**

Item#	Qty.	Item Description	Price Ea.	Total
#NWD01-V		Warrior Growth Serum Vanilla—4.5 oz	$49.95	
#NWD01-C		Warrior Growth Serum Chocolate—6 oz.	$49.95	
#NWD02-V		Warrior Milk Vanilla—16 oz.	$39.95	
#NWD02-C		Warrior Milk Chocolate—18 oz.	$39.95	
#NWD03		Warrior Stubborn Fat Burner—45 caps 500 mg	$35.95	
#NWD04		Warrior Male Performance Support—60 caps 500 mg	$39.95	
#NWD08A		Warrior Live Minerals—60 caps 880 mg	$29.95	

Or send your check or money order made out to:

Dragon Door Publications
PO Box 4381,
St. Paul, MN 55104

Shipping address (if different from address on other side of this coupon)

Name:_____

Address:_____

City:_____ State: _____

Zip:_____ Phone:_____

e-mail:_____

HANDLING AND SHIPPING CHARGES

Total amount of order add:

$00.00	to	$24.99	add	$5.00
$25.00	to	$39.99	add	$6.00
$40.00	to	$59.99	add	$7.00
$60.00	to	$99.99	add	$10.00
$100.00	to	$129.99	add	$12.00
$130.00	to	$169.99	add	$14.00
$170.00	to	$199.99	add	$16.00
$200.00	to	$299.99	add	$18.00
$300.00	and up		add	$20.00

NO COD's

Total of Goods	
Discount Amount ($10 per item)	
Shipping Charges	
MN residents add 6.5% sales tax	
Total Enclosed	

Method of payment: ___Check ___M.O.

___Mastercard ___Visa ___Discover ___Amex

Account No. _____

Expiration Date_____Date_____

Signature _____

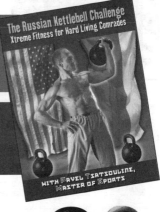
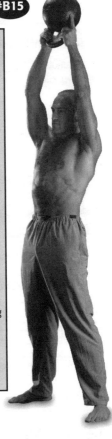
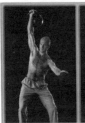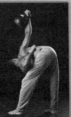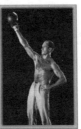

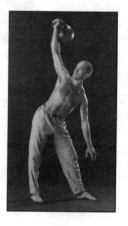

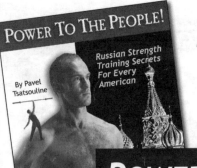

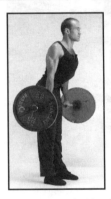

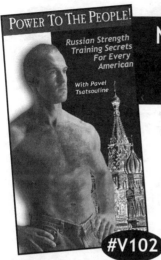

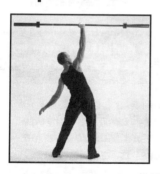
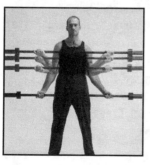

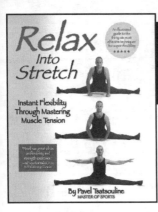

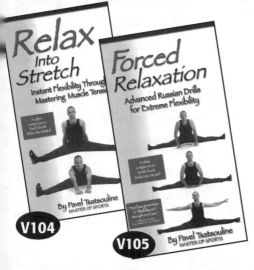

"The Do-It-Now, Fast-Start, Get-Up-and-Go, Jump-into-Action Bible for High Performance and Longer Life"

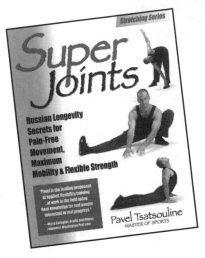

Stretching Series

Super Joints

Russian Longevity Secrets for Pain-Free Movement, Maximum Mobility & Flexible Strength

"Pavel is the leading proponent of applied flexibility training at work in the field today. Real knowledge for real people interested in real progress."
—Marty Gallagher, health and fitness columnist WashingtonPost.com

Pavel Tsatsouline
MASTER OF SPORTS

Super Joints
Russian Longevity Secrets for Pain-Free Movement, Maximum Mobility & Flexible Stength

With Pavel Tsatsouline
#B16   **$34.95**
8 1/2" x 11" Paperback
130 pages - Over 100 photos and illustrations

You have a choice in life. You can sputter and stumble and creak your way along in a process of painful, slow decline—or you can take charge of your health and become a human dynamo.

And there is no better way to insure a long, pain-free life than performing the right daily combination of joint mobility and strength-flexibility exercises.

In *Super Joints*, Russian fitness expert Pavel Tsatsouline shows you exactly how to quickly achieve and maintain peak joint health—and then use it to improve every aspect of your physical performance.

Only the foolish would deliberately ignore the life-saving and life-enhancing advice Pavel offers in *Super Joints*. Why would anyone willingly subject themselves to a life of increasing pain, degeneration and decrepitude? But for an athlete, a dancer, a martial artist or any serious performer, *Super Joints* could spell the difference between greatness and mediocrity.

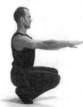

Discover:

- The twenty-eight most valuable drills for youthful joints and a stronger stretch
- How to save your joints and prevent or reduce arthritis
- The one-stop care-shop for your inner Tin Man— how to give your nervous system a tune up, your joints a lube-job and your energy a recharge
- What it takes to go from cruise control to full throttle: The One Thousand Moves Morning Recharge—Amosov's "bigger bang" calisthenics complex for achieving heaven-on earth in 25 minutes
- How to make your body feel better than you can remember— active flexibility fosporting prowess and fewer injuries
- The amazing Pink Panther technique that may add a couple of feet to your stretch the first time you do it

Complete and mail with full payment to:
Dragon Door Publications, P.O. Box 4381, St. Paul, MN 55104

SHIP TO: *(Street address for delivery)* **B**

Name_____

Street_____

City_____

State _____ Zip _____

Email_____

SOLD TO: A

Name_____

Street_____

City_____

State _____ Zip _____

Day phone*_____
* Important for clarifying questions on orders

Item #	Qty.	Item Description	Item Price	A or B	Total

HANDLING AND SHIPPING CHARGES

Total Amount of Order	Add:
$00.00 to $24.99	add $5.00
$25.00 to $39.99	add $6.00
$40.00 to $59.99	add $7.00
$60.00 to $99.99	add $10.00
$100.00 to $129.99	add $12.00
$130.00 to $169.99	add $14.00
$170.00 to $199.99	add $16.00
$200.00 to $299.99	add $18.00
$300.00 and up	add $20.00

NO COD's

Canada &
Mexico add $8.00.
All other
countries
triple U.S. charges.

Total of Goods _____

Shipping Charges _____

Rush Charges _____

MN residents add 6.5 % sales tax _____

Total Enclosed _____

Method of Payment ☐ Check ☐ M.O. ☐ Mastercard ☐ Visa ☐ Discover ☐ Diners Club ☐ Amex

Account No. *(Please indicate all the numbers on your credit card)*   EXPIRATION DATE

☐☐☐☐ ☐☐☐☐ ☐☐☐☐ ☐☐☐☐   ☐☐/☐☐

DAY PHONE ( )_____ SIGNATURE_____ DATE_____

NOTE: We ship all orders by UPS Ground, unless you request US Mail. Foreign orders are sent by Air Printed Matter. Credit card or International M.O. only. For rush processing of your order, add an additional $10.00 per address. Available on money order & harge card orders only.   Errors and omissions excepted. Prices subject to change without notice.

Customer Service Questions?
Please call us between 9 am - 5 pm (CST) Monday - Friday at (651) 487-2180 or leave us a message any time for a prompt response.

100% One-Year Risk-Free Guarantee.
If you are not completely satisfied with any product-for any reason, no matter how long after you received it-we'll be happy to give you a prompt exchange, credit, or refund, as you wish. Simply return your purchase to us, and please let us know why you were dissatisfied-it will help us to provide better products and services in the future. *Shipping and handling fees are non-refundable.*

Telephone Orders For faster service you may place your orders by calling Toll Free 24 hours a day, 7 days a week, 365 days per year. When you call, please have your credit card ready